INCREASE YO

Increase your sex drive

DR SARAH BREWER

Thorsons
An Imprint of HarperCollins*Publishers*

Thorsons
An Imprint of HarperCollins*Publishers*
77–85 Fulham Palace Road,
Hammersmith, London W6 8JB

Published by Thorsons 1999
10 9 8 7 6 5 4 3 2 1

A catalogue record for this book
is available from the British Library

ISBN 0 7225 3697 6

Printed and bound in Great Britain by
Caledonian International Book Manufacturing Ltd, Glasgow

Dedication

This book is dedicated to the millions of men and women currently struggling to understand and cope with their under-active sex drive. May the information contained in these pages speed them towards recovery. If you would like to share your experience of the plans in this book – and how quickly they worked for you – please either write to me c/o Thorsons, or via e-mail: drsarah@compuserve.com.

Acknowledgements

Many thanks to everyone who helped me to compile this book, especially Howard Thomas of Life Plus Europe, Ltd, who provided a mountain of invaluable herbal information for Chapter 9.

And, as always, thanks to my family – Nina, Richard and Saxon – for providing vital back-up support throughout the long hours I spend holed up in my study.

My agent, Serafina Clarke, also deserves credit for her unfailing enthusiasm and professionalism.

Contents

There was a young lady from Spain
Who liked a bit now and again
Not 'now-and-again' but 'Now!' and 'Again!'
And again-and-again-and-again.

Foreword

Low sex drive is common, and affects up to one fifth the population at any one time. Few people are aware that there are many effective ways to overcome the problem. In researching this book, I was astounded by the vast range of prosexual substances – vitamins, minerals, herbs, essential oils and even drugs – that have a profound and beneficial effect on libido.

If low sex drive is not a problem for you or your partner, it is not necessary to do anything about it. If low sex drive is having a profound effect on your life, relationship and wellbeing however, this book will help you overcome it. As well as detailing all the self-help measures available, a number of programmes are suggested at the back of the book to help different people with different problems boost their sex drive.

In the majority of cases, these programmes will work. Where they do not, it is important to seek medical advice. Do not be embarrassed to seek help – your doctor deals with similar problems every day, and there is nothing you can tell him or her that will shock them. A low sex drive that does not respond to treatment may be linked with a hormonal balance which needs medical assessment and treatment. In cases where the programmes do not work and medical investigations are normal, then referral to a trained psychosexual or relationship therapist will help to untangle the web of factors that are contributing to your lowered libido.

It would be irresponsible not to point out that a renewed interest in sex should not be indulged at the expense of overall health. If you are unfit, do not take part in vigorous sexual activity until you are able to cope with the brisk exercise it entails. It is no good rediscovering your sex drive if you then immediately succumb to a heart attack. Similarly, it is vital to only indulge in safer sex to minimise your risk of acquiring a sexually transmissible disease.

Introduction

Sex drive, or libido, is normally the second strongest urge in humans, after sleep. Everyone has a different sex drive, however, and this can vary significantly from person to person and from time to time. As long as you and your partner are both happy with the frequency at which you make love, you should consider your sex drive to be normal for you. Too often however, one partner develops a low sex drive, while that of their partner remains unchanged. This frequently causes problems in a relationship, with the partner having a lower libido feeling pressurized, and the other feeling neglected or unloved.

Loss of sex drive is incredibly common, and is now the biggest single reason for consulting a sex therapist. In various surveys, loss of libido has been found to affect:

- 20% of the population at any one time
- 30% of middle-aged women
- 45% of men with prostate symptoms
- 60% of stressed executives
- 72% of postmenopausal women
- 80% of new mothers and those who are breastfeeding.

A recent survey confirmed that one in five adults of all ages were dissatisfied with their sex life. One of the commonest problems was lack of desire – either in the person asked or in their partner – resulting in them not having enough sex as often as they would wish.

Luckily, a low sex drive can usually be corrected through a number of dietary and lifestyle changes, as well as taking one or more of the many prosexual supplements available.

Sex and health

A normal sex drive is desirable as your sexual health and general wellbeing are closely linked. Just as the more healthy you are the more you are likely to have sex, increased sexual vitality is also beneficial for mind, body and spirit. People with a healthy sex life commonly feel more alive than those who do not.

The benefits of regular sex have been suggested through the ages. In ancient China, the flow of sexual energy round the body was believed to form the basis of physical, emotional and spiritual wellbeing, and channelling sexual energy was considered the key to immortality. Herbal aphrodisiacs and erotic arts were therefore used extensively – not to increase simple pleasure in sex, but as a means to improved general health and longevity.

This concept is now embraced by Chinese medicine, in which sexual energy is viewed as a manifestation of constitutional essence, or *Jing*. *Jing* is stored in the kidneys and is responsible for the cycles that allow growth, reproduction and development. If *Jing* is excessively depleted, it is believed to lead to premature ageing and recurrent ill health. In the West, sensuality and relaxation are often viewed separately and the balance between them neglected, especially by those under pressure for the more stressed you are, the lower your sex drive will become. Chinese medicine sees this as nature's way of conserving *Jing* and considers it a sign of imbalance and ill-health.

Many practitioners of Chinese medicine recommend that sex is followed by a period of relaxation to allow sexual energy and libido to rejuvenate. The quality of *Jing* can also be strengthened by activating an area below the umbilicus known as the *Tan Tien* (seat of the *Jing*) through breathing exercises, adjusting body posture and focused visualization (*see Chapter 12*). When the *Tan Tien* is activated, a vibration is felt in the area and it may also become warmer. Interestingly there are many parallels between *Jing* and the hormone, dehydroepiandrostenedione (DHEA) – not least the fact that DHEA is produced just above the kidneys in the adrenal glands. DHEA is the master sex hormone whose levels rise during sex to three or five times higher than normal. DHEA has a number of beneficial actions, including a prosexual effect and the potential to prolong life (*see Chapters 2 and 8*).

The Greek physician, Galen, wrote in the second century AD that sexual abstinence was the direct cause of hysteria, while in the 1940s, psychoanalyst Wilhelm Reich advocated an orgasm a day for optimum health.

Researchers have now found many beneficial effects of indulging in regular sex. The 'little death' as the French call sexual climax, may help to postpone the big death that is on everyone's agenda in the future. A study involving nearly 1000 men in Caerphilly, UK, found that the risk of death at any age in men with a high orgasmic frequency (twice a week or more) was half that of men with a low orgasmic frequency (less than once a month). The authors concluded that sexual activity seems to have a protective effect on men's health – although it is possible that the association could be the other way round: people who are ill are less likely to have sex than those who are healthy.

Weekly sex is also important for a woman's physiology and reproductive health. Regular sex can increase blood oestrogen levels, helping to protect against coronary heart disease and brittle bones (osteoporosis). This also helps to normalize an irregular menstrual cycle and reduce the symptoms of premenstrual syndrome. Sexual abstinence on the other hand has been found to lower oestrogen levels and may be linked with menstrual and menopausal problems. Research in the US involving both young, undergraduate women and older women approaching the menopause, found that those having regular sex every week (except during menstruation) tended to be more fertile. They had oestrogen levels around twice as high as those who were less sexually active. Women who only indulged in occasional sex had a high risk of severely low oestrogen levels at any age, and this can have a profound effect on quality of life at the menopause. Menopausal women having regular sex had less hot flushes and tended to age more slowly than those who did not have sex at least once a week.

Sexual activity is also good for keeping the pelvic floor muscles toned, helping to reduce the risk of stress incontinence, prolapse and for making sex more enjoyable for both partners. Sexercise also keeps muscle groups in the lower back, stomach and bottom firm.

In men, male hair growth seems to increase when sex is anticipated, probably as a result of increased testosterone activity. Testosterone levels have been found to increase during and after sex which may provide some protection against male osteoporosis and coronary heart disease, as well as improving muscle bulk and maintaining the size of the penis and testicles. Regular sex also allows men to benefit from the beneficial effects of DHEA (*see Chapters 2 and 8*) – DHEA levels rise just before orgasm and ejaculation to three to five times higher than normal, which some claim is one of the reasons that regular sex can prolong your life. Regular sex also helps to prevent congestion of the prostate gland which has been linked with an increased risk of prostatitis (inflammation of the gland).

In both men and women, levels of the hormone, oxytocin (*see Chapter 2*), peak during orgasm, having a tranquillizing effect in both men and women, helping to provide a good night's sleep. This effect is greater in males than females. Oxytocin is also the hormone that helps to bind a couple together in love, and a regular sex life will help to cement a relationship.

Another beneficial effect of sex is that it is an excellent reliever of stress and mild aches and pains. Testosterone has a painkilling action by damping down inflammation, especially in joints. Research suggests that some arthritis sufferers have less pain for up to six hours after sex. Don't make love if you have a headache however. Some evidence suggests this may re-trigger the headache every time you have an orgasm for at least six weeks afterwards – and in some cases, the effect lasts more than a year. The infamous phrase 'Not tonight, I have a headache', has some basis in reality, after all.

Like other forms of exercise, sex has been shown to improve general fitness. During sexual arousal, your body undergoes several powerful, physical changes. Your skin flushes, more energy is dissipated as heat, your pulse races to an average of 114 beats per minute (and sometimes to as high as 140 – 150 beats per minute), blood pressure rises and you breath more deeply. These changes all help to boost your metabolic rate. And that's just from thinking about sex, before you even lift a finger (or leg) to do anything about it. These changes are virtually identical to those that occur during intense exercise and can give similar health benefits. Sex increases blood oxygen levels, strengthens muscle tone and helps to keep you mentally alert. Adults are advised to exercise regularly for 20 – 30 minutes at least five times per week (and preferably every day) at a brisk rate that is enough to raise the pulse above 100 beats per minute. What better way to obtain this exercise than by making love?

A vigorous lovemaking session can burn 500 kcals per hour – equivalent to gentle jogging or moderate cycling. For the averagely active person, 30 minutes of sexual exercise (equivalent to walking briskly at 4.5 miles per hour) will burn around 200 calories – enough to lose one pound of fat every two weeks if you indulged every day.

Sex can also help to improve your strength (by building muscle bulk), stamina (by increasing muscle energy stores) and suppleness (by improving flexibility), which compares with other popular activities as follows:

Activity	Stamina	Strength	Suppleness
Cricket	*	*	**
Golf	*	*	**
Walking (ramble)	**	*	*
Missionary position	**	*	*
Downhill Skiing	**	**	**
Tennis	**	**	**
Badminton	**	**	***
Hill walking	***	**	*
Rowing	***	**	*
Skipping	***	**	**
Vigorous sex	***	**	**
Aerobics	***	**	***
Squash	***	**	***
Athletics	***	***	**
Circuit Training	***	***	***
Football	***	***	***
Jogging	****	**	**
Cycling	****	***	**
Hard swimming	****	****	****
Athletic sex	****	****	****

* = Slight effect ** = Beneficial effect *** = Very good effect
**** = Excellent effect

Contrary to popular belief, sex can even boost athletic performance. A US study tested 11 men on a treadmill, some of whom had had sexual intercourse 12 hours before. Aerobic capacity was found to be exactly the same in both groups and the researchers concluded that athletes can have intercourse without it affecting their performance. One Olympic middle-distance champion is known to have broken the world record an hour after sex, and a British runner ran a four-minute mile only 1.5 hours after making love.

When you are enjoying a healthy sex life, all aspects of life tend to take on a rosier hue. Regular sex is important for general wellbeing and quality of life. It's not the be-all and end-all of a relationship however. If a couple are happy with a low level of sexual interaction, this should not be regarded as a problem. Long-lasting partnerships are built on friendship, love, laughter, humour and shared experiences as much as on a normal sex drive. If lack of sex is causing problems however, this book contains all the information you need to help overcome the problem – either through taking natural herbal supplements, seeking advice about hormone replacement therapy, or seeking help from a psychosexual counsellor.

How to Use this Book

The easiest way to use this book to increase your sex drive is to turn to Chapter 15: *Boost your sex drive* (page 245) and to read the individually tailored plan most suited to your circumstances. You can then go back to the relevant parts of the book to read more about the vitamin, mineral, herbal, aromatherapy and homeopathic supplements recommended for your particular time of life. This approach lets you start your libido-boosting programme straight away without waiting to read the rest of the book first.

1

What is a normal sex drive?

The sex drive, or libido, is a powerful directing force that has a profound effect on human behaviour. The term libido was first used by the psychoanalyst, Sigmund Freud, to signify the instinctive psychosexual energy that is present in everyone from birth. He suggested that during the first year of life, the libido is focused on the mouth during the oral phase of development. During the second year, libido shifted to the anal area, while between the ages of three and six, the libido moves to the genitals. Freud claimed that psychiatric illness was the direct result of a libido that was misdirected or frustrated. The term libido is now used more generally however, to describe the basic desire for sex, which, after the need for sleep, is usually the strongest urge experienced by humans.

Sexologists describe two main types of sex drive:

- the aggressive, testosterone-dominant, physical libido, in which there is an outward drive to find a sexual mate, and
- the receptive, oestrogen-dominant, psychological libido, in which there is a passive willingness to receive the sexual overtures of a potential mate.

Men are said to reach their peak physical sex drive in their teens, while their psychological sex drive peaks after the age of 50 when testosterone levels fall. Women are said to reach their physical sexual peak in their thirties or forties while their psychological sex drive reaches its maximum in their 50s, at the same time as that of males.

Sex drive varies considerably from person to person however, and also from time to time. Some people are driven by a powerful libido that fuels sexual activity at least once a day. For others, sex drive is naturally low-key and is satisfied by sexual intimacy occurring less than once a month.

An Esquire/MORI Survey of 800 men, aged 18–45 years, with and without regular partners (figures rounded to nearest integer so add up to 101%) showed that:

- 2% had intercourse more than once a day or at least every day.
- 11% had sex 4 to 6 times a week.
- 33% 2 to 3 times per week.
- 19% once a week.
- 11% once a fortnight.
- 7% once a month.
- 13% – less than once a month.
- 5% of non-virgin males were not actively indulging at the moment.

The Hite Report on Male Sexuality, 10 years earlier, found that 27% of men made love once a week and 12% just once a fortnight.

Another UK survey found that:

- 40% of adult couples make love more than three times per week.
- 35% make love once or twice a week.
- 15% make love two to three times per month.
- 9% of couples make love less than this or not at all.

The large, US National Survey of Families and Households (1995) involved over 13,000 people and found that the average couple had sex an average of 10.4 times per month. The rate was highest where the male partner was aged 19–24 (14.9 times per month) and lowest in the over 60s (2.3 times per month). The survey also found that the frequency at which a person makes love seems to depend on three main factors:

- The length of time in a particular relationship – around 50% of couples together for under three years made love more than three times per week. After four years together, only 25% kept this up. After five years in a relationship, sexual activity fell each year by an average of 0.9 times per month.
- The overall health of the male – those in excellent health made love an average of 10.93 times per month compared with 9.41 times for those who felt their health was only fair or poor.
- The age of the female sex partner – as she grew older, a couple were likely to make love less each month – but where the woman was much older than the male, the couple were likely to make love more than average.

Other surveys have found that combined income is also important – the more a person earns, the less likely they are to have sex regularly due to stress and physical exhaustion.

By the time you reach your late 30s, you will probably be having sex less often than in your youth as you are more likely to be settled into a long-term relationship. The number of times a couple have intercourse halves after the first year or two they have been together.

Sex drive usually declines with age as an inevitable result of lower levels of sex hormones and some loss of vitality. Some research suggests that the average number of orgasms experienced annually by both men and women varies with age as follows:

Age	Number of orgasms per year
20	104
30	121
40	84
50	52
60	35
70	22

The time taken to reach orgasm and the time for sex drive to recover (refractory period) after ejaculation also varies with age in men. One in five males in their 20s–30s reach orgasm within a minute of starting to make love – 62% within five minutes. Sex drive recovers quickly – usually within five to ten minutes of orgasm.

By the age of 45, testosterone levels have fallen significantly so that sex drive recovers more slowly – around an hour after orgasm.

By the age of 70, testosterone levels are approaching their lowest ebb. Sex drive may take 24 hours to recover after orgasm and erectile difficulties become increasingly common.

Research shows that sexual interest falls off more rapidly in women than men between the ages of 50 to 60 years. By the age of 70, half of all women admit to having little interest in sex, compared with only 10% of men at the same age.

According to a recent survey, women aged 20 – 29 made love around five times per month while women aged 55 – 59 made love twice a month or less. Half of all women in this age group admitted to not having sex at all in the previous month.

Whatever your age, however, it is possible to successfully boost your sex drive within just a few weeks – most people will respond to a simple self-help programme involving massage, aromatherapy, multivitamins and minerals plus herbal supplements. Where these do not help, hormone replacement therapy or psychosexual therapy will usually resolve the problem. The following chapters show you how.

2

How your sex drive
is controlled

Sex drive, or libido, is controlled through complex interactions
between:

- Sex hormones (DHEA, FSH, LH, pregnenolone.
  androstenedione, testosterone, oestrogen and progesterone).
- Metabolic hormones (cortisol, growth hormone, adrenaline,
  prolactin, oxytocin, thyroxine, PEA, vasopressin and various
  releasing hormones from the hypothalamus).
- Brain neurotransmitters (e.g. serotonin, dopamine.
  acetylcholine, gamma-aminobutyric acid (GABA),
  noradrenaline).
- Pheromones.
- Psychological stimuli (sight, imagination).
- Physical stimuli (taste, smell, touch).
- Cultural customs/inhibitions – some native tribesmen
  believe, for example, that if they don't have sex every day,
  their penis will stop working.

These interactions are further modified by external factors such as
levels of stress, exercise, drug and alcohol intakes, smoking habits,
general health, fatigue, diet and even the amount of sunlight you are
exposed to.

The desire for sex is regulated in appetite centres found in the limbic system and hypothalamus of the brain. The control centre for male sexual behaviour is now known to be in the anterior hypothalamus, while the sexual centre for women is in the region of the ventromedial nucleus. The chemicals which have the most profound effect on control of sex drive are reviewed below:

DHEA (Dehydroepiandrosterone)

DHEA is often described as the master sex hormone. It starts being made in large quantities at puberty and levels peak in the early twenties. Between the ages of 30 to 50, the amount produced falls slowly by around 80% from an average of 30mg in youth to just 6mg in later life. It is now known that high DHEA levels are linked with the highest sex drives, so falling levels of DHEA partly account for reduced sex drive with increasing age.

DHEA levels also rise just before orgasm to three to five times higher than normal, which some suggest is the reason why regular sex can prolong your life. Exercise – like sex – increases DHEA levels temporarily but only if it is consistent and sustained. You need to exercise vigorously for 30 minutes a day for one month before significant increases in DHEA levels occur. (*For more information about DHEA, see Chapter 8*).

Oxytocin

Oxytocin is a hormone secreted by the pituitary gland. It stimulates ejection of milk during breastfeeding but also plays a role in contraction of muscles in the penis, uterus and vagina during orgasm. Oxytocin has been described as the hormone of mother love, the hormone of monogamy and the hormonal equivalent of super-glue as it is important for binding relationships together. Oxytocin levels rise whenever you think of someone you fancy and surge even higher when you are in close enough proximity to touch them. Having sex sends oxytocin levels soaring to five times higher than normal. From an emotional point of view, the rise in oxytocin levels that occurs with skin-to-skin contact and at the point of climax, helps you bond with your partner and also makes you feel drowsy so you enjoy a more refreshing and restorative night's sleep after having made love.

PEA (phenylethylamine)

PEA is sometimes referred to as the molecular basis for love. PEA is chemically related to amphetamine and is responsible for the initial feelings of swooning, walking on air and loss of appetite that accompany falling in love. PEA produces a pleasant euphoria and is also released during orgasm to help intensify the sensation. It seems to be mildly addictive and, as levels also increase when eating chocolate, may account for the more-ish nature of both sex and chocolate.

Oestrogen

Oestrogen is a collection of three female hormones: oestradiol (the most powerful oestrogen), oestrone and oestriol (the weakest) that play an important role in female sexuality. Small quantities are also present in males and play a role in their sexual behaviour. When oestrogen is given to men (for example as part of the treatment of prostate cancer), it has a prosexual effect. (*For more information about oestrogen, see Chapter 8*).

Testosterone

Testosterone is known as the male hormone, although it is also present in women in significant amounts and plays an important role in helping to control female sex drive – probably by interacting with the

brain chemical, dopamine. Testosterone is responsible for male characteristics such as hairiness, muscle development and baldness and
there may be some truth in the old wives' tale that bald men are
sexier. Men with the highest testosterone levels are certainly more
sexually active than those with the lowest levels. Research shows that
men with the lowest testosterone levels are more faithful however,
being more likely to get married and to successfully stay married. This
may be because low testosterone levels make men more docile, less
aggressive, better humoured and more home loving. In a study of over
4000 American males, it was found that husbands with high testosterone levels were 43% more likely to get divorced and 38% more
likely to have extramarital affairs than men with lower levels. They
were also 50% less likely to get married in the first place.

Castration (removal of the testicles) is eventually followed by a
reduction in sexual activity, but this may not be for several years. In
many cases, sexual activity does not peter out altogether. This may be
due to an increased output of testosterone from the adrenal glands,
which usually only provide 5% of circulating testosterone levels.

In males who do lose their sex drive and ability to have erections
as a result of low testosterone levels, testosterone replacement
therapy can effectively reverse these changes and restore sexual
activity to its former level. It will not have a significant positive effect
on sex drive in men whose testosterone levels are normal, however.

Testosterone and related androgens also play an important role in
controlling sex drive in women, and are produced in small amounts
by the ovaries and the adrenal glands. Female sex drive may
increase at certain times of the menstrual cycle, especially midcycle
when levels of oestrogen and testosterone peak. This increase in
sexual desire is designed by evolution to maximize the chance of
fertilization at ovulation.

New research has found that a man's testerone levels, and his
libido, is closely linked to the length of his ring finger. Men whose

third fingers are much longer than their index finger tend to have higher testosterone levels and a higher sex drive than those whose ring and index fingers are of a similar length. In women, a longer index finger is associated with higher levels of oestrogen and luteinizing hormone.

The shape, size and symmetry of the hands and whether or not the left and right hands are closely matched, is also linked to a higher fertility in men and women, and a higher sperm count in males. This is thought to be because genes involved in hand development in the womb are also involved in determining development of the ovaries or testicles. (*For more information about testosterone, see Chapter 8*).

Dopamine

Dopamine is the brain chemical (neurotransmitter) that drives the anticipation and desire for any pleasurable activity. It produces feelings of enthusiasm and excitement, lifts a low mood, increases feelings of pleasure and has a powerful ability to boost sex drive and make orgasm easier to achieve. It is closely linked with the regulation of testosterone production, and low levels of dopamine result in a low sex drive. Drugs that increase levels of dopamine have a marked stimulatory effect on libido. (*For more information see Chapter 14*).

Serotonin

Serotonin is a brain chemical that is linked with appetite and satiation for both food and sex. High levels of serotonin damp down your sex drive (and appetite for food), the ability to achieve orgasm, and can also induce passive, sluggish behaviour. In low levels, serotonin stimulates desire for both food and sex and also promotes aggressive behaviour. Low levels make it easier to reach sexual climax.

Pheromones

Pheromones are volatile chemicals that are subconsciously detected in the nose to have a profound effect on human sexuality. These powerful chemicals (e.g. androstenol and androsterone) are secreted in sweat and vaginal secretions. Women are especially sensitive to male pheromones when they are ovulating, and also produce their most powerful pheromones at this time of the menstrual cycle. In a double-blind* study investigating male reactions to female vaginal pheromones, men were exposed to one of three vaginal secretions (premenstrual, menstrual, ovulatory) or water, through an inhaler, then asked to judge the attractiveness of women in five photos. The men exposed to vaginal secretions gave higher attraction ratings, as compared to men exposed to only water. The ovulatory secretions produced the highest ratings, and also increased the men's testosterone levels. (*For more information about pheromones, see chapter 5*).

Sexual Memory

Sex is a basic survival activity in which the pleasurable sensations involved originate in a relatively primitive part of the brain that has little capacity to store memory. As a result, it is difficult to remember feelings of pleasure – just as it is difficult to remember the sensations involved in pain. The memory of sexual pleasure therefore fades quickly, and this can be a major problem with low sex drive. Because you can't remember how wonderful sex feels, there is little impetus to experience it again. One way round this is to use your sense of smell. Smell is also activated in primitive parts of the brain and has a powerful, evocative effect on memory. Whenever you make love, use a particular, self-chosen blend of aromatherapy oils. When you

---

* A study in which neither researchers nor volunteers know which chemicals are being used.

want to boost your sex drive in the future, smell this particular aromatherapy blend again and use creative visualization (*see Chapter 12*) to help trigger memories of the sensations and feelings involved. Alternatively, imagine having sex while actually sniffing an unwashed item of your lover's clothing so you smell their secret scent (and pheromones) instead.

Having explored the main mechanisms that control a normal sex drive, the following chapter looks at the many factors that can have a negative effect on libido, and which can reduce or wipe it out altogether.

For more information on how sex drive is controlled, read *Why We Love and Lust – How our sex hormones influence our relationships* by Dr Theresa Crenshaw (*see Resources*).

3

Why sex drive can fail

Everyone's definition of a low sex drive will vary. For some, sex drive will be low if they only indulge in sex once a week, while others may not consider their drive low until they are only indulging once a fortnight or less. When sex drive fails completely however, the effects are indisputable. Sufferers will experience a global loss of interest in sex and will rarely, if ever, think about sex, have erotic fantasies or dreams, or have any desire to seek intimate contact or sexual pleasure. They will also have a similar disinterest in masturbation.

Loss of sex drive can occur for a number of different reasons, of which the most common include:

- familiarity
- lack of exercise
- overweight
- low self-esteem and poor body image
- stress
- lack of sleep
- poor diet
- excess alcohol
- smoking
- drugs

- pregnancy
- breastfeeding
- anxiety
- depression
- pain
- hysterectomy
- female menopause
- male menopause
- prostate problems
- hypogonadism (underactive ovaries or testicles)
- prolactinoma (prolactin-secreting tumour of the pituitary gland.
- chronic disease
- previous sexual abuse
- relationship problems
- lack of sunshine
- cultural influences

These factors, and the way they affect your sex drive, are explored individually below.

Familiarity

Once you are happily settled in a loving, long-term relationship, the sensual thrills that accompanied the first flush of love will damp down. Once the passionate, honeymoon phase is over, lovemaking often becomes less exciting because you are familiar with your lover's body and their tried, tested (and repeated) techniques. If both partners in the relationship are happy with the status quo, there is no problem. If one develops a sex drive that is lower than their partner feels comfortable with, this will usually cause relationship difficulties. Try to keep interest in sex alive by experimenting with different positions and techniques, and varying the time and place of lovemaking so your love life does not become stale.

Lack of exercise

General unfitness and lack of exercise can lower sex drive through several effects on metabolism and hormone balance. In particular, it can lower levels of DHEA (dehydroepiandrosterone – *see Chapters 2 and 8*). Regular, brisk exercise for 30 minutes a day can help to boost DHEA secretion. This level of exercise needs to be sustained for a continuous effect however, and is most marked after regularly exercising for at least a month. Exercise also stimulates release of phenylethylamine (PEA – *see Chapter 2*), which helps to intensify orgasm. Increasing your overall fitness level will help to boost your sex drive. Don't overdo exercise however – over-exercising for as little as two weeks can lower testosterone levels by a third. These effects can take three months to return to normal when over-training is stopped.

Overweight

Researchers estimate that one in two of the Western population are now overweight (10% above their ideal weight), and a further one in five are obese (20% above ideal weight). Being overweight or obese frequently leads to sluggishness, low energy levels, lack of self-esteem and low sex drive. Excess consumption of carbohydrate causes raised levels of serotonin in the brain which also has a strong, libido-lowering effect (*see Chapter 2*). In contrast, losing excess weight can boost your sex drive. Weight loss reduces levels of serotonin in the brain which helps to boost sex drive as body image and self esteem improve.

Low self-esteem and poor body image

One of the most inhibiting factors when it comes to making love is lack of confidence in your body shape. Women who feel their breasts are the wrong size, their tummy too big, or their thighs or bottom too large have been known to go to extraordinary lengths in order to avoid sex. In one survey, 25% of women were unhappy with the size of their breasts, over 40% were unhappy with their bottoms, thighs or stomachs, and this was felt to have a negative affect on sexuality. Taking exercise, getting fit and losing excess weight will improve self esteem, but it is important to learn to accept and even love your body as it is now (*see Chapter 12*).

Stress

Stress is one of the commonest causes of loss of libido, along with overwork, tiredness and lack of sleep. The adrenal glands usually produce around 5% of circulating sex hormones such as oestrogen and testosterone. When under stress, the adrenal glands produce increased amounts of cortisol and adrenaline instead, and the adrenal boost to sex drive switches off.

Stress significantly reduces levels of DHEA in the brain, and also decreases secretion of gonadotrophin releasing hormone (GnRH) the master hormone that kick-starts the ovaries and testicles to produce oestrogen and testosterone. As a result, oestrogen and testosterone levels will fall. One of the most significant causes of reduced sex drive in stressed individuals however, is increased secretion of prolactin hormone which occurs in surges during times of stress, to turn the libido off.

Unfortunately, stress is common. A survey by *Men's Health* magazine found that stress was the biggest concern for male readers. A quarter of men had taken time off work to escape stress – an average of six days per year – and one in three admitted to taking time off work by pretending to be ill. The major sources of stress were:

- work itself   79%
- money worries   45%

- relationships   36%
- health problems   12%
- unemployment   11%

Reducing stress levels will help to boost sex drive in both men and women. You should also aim to avoid coffee, strong tea, caffeinated drinks, cigarettes and alcohol when you are under stress as these can all make the problem worse. Follow a wholefood diet and take a good multi-vitamin and mineral supplement. Relaxation techniques such as meditation, massage, having a warm aromatherapy bath by candlelight and taking time out to rest and relax are essential. Interestingly, men are more likely to make love to relax than women.

Lack of sleep

Lack of sleep, due to working long hours, commuting, shift work, jet lag, or being woken by a baby can have a serious damping effect on sex drive. It is estimated that 60% of adults experience some degree of insomnia on a regular basis, with difficulty falling asleep, waking in the middle of the night and not being able to get back to sleep, sleeping fitfully, or waking up still feeling tired because sleep was not restorative. Tips to help you wake up feeling better include:

- Avoid taking naps during the day as this will make it more difficult to sleep at night.
- Take regular exercise, but avoid strenuous exercise late in the evening as this will keep you awake.
- Follow a healthy, wholefood diet with plenty of complex carbohydrates (e.g. cereals, bread, pasta) and fruit and vegetables for vitamins and minerals. Try to eat your evening meal before 7pm and resist late night snacks, especially of rich food.

- Avoid over-indulgence in substances that interfere with sleep such as caffeine (coffee, tea, chocolate, colas) nicotine and alcohol – although alcohol may help you fall asleep, you are likely to have a disturbed sleep once the drugged effect has worn off.

- Take time to unwind from the stresses of the day before going to bed – read a book, listen to soothing music or have a candlelit bath.

- A warm, milky drink just before going to bed will help you to relax – hot milk with cinnamon or nutmeg is better than chocolate drinks that contain some caffeine.

- Don't drink too much fluid in the evening – a full bladder is guaranteed to disturb your rest.

- Develop the habit of going to bed at a regular time each night and getting up at the same time each morning.

- Set a bedtime routine such as checking house security, brushing your teeth, bathing and setting the alarm clock to set the mood for sleep.

- Make sure your bed is comfortable, and your bedroom warm, dark and quiet – noise and excessive cold or heat will keep you awake. A temperature of 18 – 24°C is ideal.

- If you can't sleep, don't lie there tossing and turning. Get up and read or watch the television for a while. If you are worried about something, write down all the things on your mind and promise yourself you will deal with them in the morning, when you are feeling fresher. When you feel sleepy, go back to bed and try again. If sleep does not come within 15 minutes, get up and repeat this process.

- Preserve your bedroom as a place for sleep (and sex) – don't use it for eating, working or watching television.

Poor diet

It is estimated that only one in ten people get all the micronutrients they need from their food. Lack of vitamins, minerals and essential fatty acids can cause hormone imbalances and have a profound effect on libido. Following a wholefood diet, not skipping meals, and taking a good multi vitamin and mineral supplement (providing around 100% of the recommended daily amount of as many micronutrients as possible) plus evening primrose oil can help to boost your sex drive. Eating plants rich in phytoestrogens can also help (*see Chapter 7*).

Excess alcohol

In small quantities, alcohol is an aphrodisiac – but only for women, it seems. After drinking two units of alcohol, female testosterone levels rise steeply one to two hours later. This effect is greatest around the time of ovulation. Alcohol does not produce the same testosterone surge in men. Unfortunately, in larger quantities alcohol goes on to lower oestrogen levels and female libido, and excessive intake can lead to loss of vaginal secretions, menstrual problems and lowered fertility. In men, any quantity of alcohol can reduce production of testosterone and hasten its conversion to oestrogen in the liver, leading to lowered sperm counts and decreased sex drive. As much as 40% of male subfertility has been blamed on just a moderate intake of alcohol alone. Excessive intakes of alcohol in males can lead to impotence, shrunken testicles, a reduction in penis size and loss of pubic hair (male hypogonadism, see below). The intakes that can trigger these problems vary from person to person, depending on how your metabolism handles alcohol and how much exercise you take. Sensible drinking levels are no more than 21 units per week for women, and 28 units per week for men. Weekly intakes of over 35 units for women and 50 units for men are considered dangerous.

Stopping drinking can improve sperm counts and increase both male and female sex drive within 3 months. Milk thistle (*see page 148*) can help to protect liver cells from the poisonous effects of alcohol and may help to boost testosterone levels where they have been lowered by excess alcohol intake.

Smoking

Smoking cigarettes lowers oestrogen levels in women – enough to bring on the menopause two to three years earlier than in non-smokers – and has a long-term detrimental effect on sex drive. In men, smoking cigarettes lowers testosterone levels. Stopping smoking, or at least cutting down, can significantly boost your sex drive.

Men who smoke have an increased risk of low sex drive and erectile problems. A study of over 300 male smokers measured penile rigidity during nocturnal erections and found a clear, inverse relationship between rigidity and the number of cigarettes smoked each day. The herbal remedy, oats, is useful when trying to stop smoking as it has both a prosexual action and an ability to help overcome addictions such as to nicotine.

Drugs

Many commonly prescribed drugs (and some illicit drugs) have a negative effect on sex drive. Doctors now accept that at least 150 medications can affect sexual function in some people. The most common culprits are:

- drugs used to treat heart and blood pressure problems, especially betablockers (e.g. propranolol, atenolol, metoprolol, guanethidine, bethanidine, hydralazine, methyldopa); diuretics (e.g. bendrofluazide, chlorthalidone, spironolactone) and digoxin.

- tranquillizers (sleeping tablets, anti-anxiety medications) especially the benzodiazepines (e.g. diazepam, temazepam, lorazepam)
- antidepressants – including selective serotonin reuptake inhibitors (SSRIs) such as Prozac (fluoxetine) and tricyclic antidepressants (e.g. amitriptyline). These can significantly reduce sex drive, cause erectile dysfunction in at least 40% of men and make orgasm difficult to achieve (and of reduced intensity) in 30% of adults taking them. Other antidepressants such as trazodone, viloxazine, fluvoxamine, and nefazodone are less likely to affect sex drive
- some anti-ulcer drugs, especially cimetidine
- corticosteroid drugs (e.g. prednisolone) and anabolic steroids
- some antihistamines (e.g. diphenhydramine, phenyl-propanolamine) many of which are also available over-the-counter
- oral contraceptives – especially progestogenic Pills that both reduce vaginal secretions and lower DHEA levels. Progestogen-only contraceptives (e.g. mini-Pill, implants, depot injections) can significantly reduce sex drive by reducing testosterone levels. One type of pill prescribed to women with acne or unwanted hair contains cyproterone, an anti-androgen that blocks the effects of testosterone and may therefore reduce libido significantly
- some cholesterol-lowering drugs which reduce production of pregnenolone
- some drugs used to treat prostate problems (e.g. finasteride, cyproterone)
- many drugs used to treat cancer
- opiates
- some antipsychotic drugs (e.g. chlorpromazine, haloperidol)

If you think your low sex drive is linked with a medication you are taking, it is worth asking your doctor if it is possible to switch to another drug or to change the dose you are taking. Do not stop taking your medication except under medical supervision, however.

Pregnancy

Sex drive can go up, go down or remain the same during pregnancy – every woman, and every pregnancy is different and does not seem to relate to the hormone changes occurring at the time. Psychological influences play a large part, as does increased blood flow to the genital area, increased lubrication and the fact that orgasm is usually easier to achieve and more intense. If low sex drive occurs, this is often linked with physical exhaustion, especially during the last three months – a time when levels of the libido-neutralizing hormone, prolactin, are also increasing. Loss of sex drive is not inevitable during pregnancy however as high levels of oestrogen and progesterone moderate the effect of prolactin. There are occasions when sex should be avoided during pregnancy, so follow the instructions of your midwife or doctors. The father-to-be will often also find his sex drive goes down. This may relate to fear of harming the baby, finding the pregnant shape less appealing, or may possibly result from changes in his female partner's pheromones.

Postnatal sex drive

Many women and their partners assume the female sex drive will quickly return to normal after having a baby. This is not always the case, however, especially in women who continue to breastfeed. High levels of the prolactin hormone, which are needed for initial production of milk, occur at this time, and have a significant damping effect on ardour and can cause sex drive to disappear altogether. This is one of nature's ways of minimizing the chance that the mother becomes pregnant again while her newborn is still highly dependent. This is an inevitable and predictable effect, although few pregnant women are warned about it. If the new mother accepts the advances of her partner however, she will still be able to reach and enjoy orgasm as usual – it is just her libido which is temporarily reduced. After childbirth, prolactin levels return to normal, non-pregnant levels within eight days if the infant is not suckled. Breast-feeding – which is by far the healthiest option for both you and your baby (unless you are HIV positive), – causes prolactin levels to stay high at first. There is no need to stop breastfeeding just to retrieve your libido, however. You just need a little patience. Even with pro-longed breastfeeding, prolactin levels slowly return to normal after you have been nursing for more than three months, so that breast-feeding continues with prolactin levels that are in the normal range. In one survey, a quarter of women interviewed a year after giving birth said they enjoyed sex more now than they did before conceiving their baby.

Other factors that may affect postnatal sex drive include being sore – especially if you have had stitches – fearing that you are too big (either vaginally or overweight), low self-esteem, anxiety about coping with the baby, fear of further pregnancy, being totally absorbed in the baby, conflict between working or not working, having difficulty reconciling your role as both a mother and a lover, and postnatal depression. If low sex drive is linked with postnatal depression, you must seek medical help from your doctor, midwife or health visitor immediately.

Anxiety

Anxiety is common, and affects at least 15% of the population, with 5% regularly suffering from panic attacks. Anxiety can lead to physical tiredness, emotional exhaustion and loss of sex drive.

Breathing exercises, behaviour therapy, counselling and alternative therapies such as homeopathy, hypnotherapy, yoga or meditation will usually help.

Depression

Depression affects at least 5% of the population at any one time and is two to three times more common in women than men. The lifetime risk of developing severe depression is around 10% for men and 25% for women. The risk amongst females may be higher because of the emotional swings occurring with premenstrual syndrome, after childbirth, and around the menopause. It is increasingly thought that the incidence in men is higher than previously believed as they are less likely to come forward and seek help. Women tend to suffer their first depressive symptoms between the ages of 35 and 55 years, 10 years earlier than men.

Loss of sex drive is one of the first symptoms to occur in depressive illness, and one of the last to recover with antidepressant therapy. If you feel your low sex drive is linked with depression, it is important to seek help from your doctor. Other symptoms of depressive illness include sleep disturbance, loss of appetite and sometimes loss of weight, low physical and mental energy levels, anxiety, tearfulness and general loss of interest in life around you. If you and your doctor together decide that you need an antidepressant medication, ask whether it is possible to have one that may stimulate your sex drive rather than damping it down further. The antidepressants that are less likely to reduce sex drive (and may even stimulate it) include trazodone, viloxazine, fluvoxamine and nefazodone.

Pain

Physical discomfort when making love can, not surprisingly, lead to lack of interest or aversion to sex, especially in females. Pain when making love may be superficial (e.g. due to vaginal thrush, allergy to spermicides, urethral sensitivity, cystitis or vaginal dryness) or deep (e.g. due to pelvic inflammatory disease, endometriosis or ovarian abnormalities including prolapse). Pain during sex is not normal, and medical advice should always be sought without delay. Sometimes using a lubricant such as KY Jelly, Replens, Senselle or Sylk is all that is needed (*see Resources*). Where appropriate, avoiding bath products and soaps may help. Gynaecological treatments such as anti-thrush therapy, antibiotics for pelvic inflammatory disease, drugs or laser treatment for endometriosis, or surgery (e.g. to stitch the ovaries back out of the line of fire of the male) are other options that may need to be considered.

Hysterectomy

Normally, during female sexual arousal, fluid is secreted into the vagina to provide lubrication, the upper third of the vagina lengthens and expands, and the uterus moves upwards. During orgasm, nerve impulses spread through various nerves to cause contraction of pelvic floor muscles and vagina. The uterus also contracts rhythmically to add to the intense sensations felt during climax.

One in three women who have had a total hysterectomy (in which the whole womb is removed) notice the loss of these uterine sensations when making love and seven out of ten find it more difficult to achieve orgasm. Although there may be no difference in your sex drive at first, studies suggest that after a year women who have had a hysterectomy have significantly less orgasms than women with an intact womb. In a few cases, the opposite is true – some women find lovemaking more enjoyable and orgasm more intense after the operation, especially if they were previously in a lot of pain.

A study in which ultrasound probes recorded what happened during intercourse in women found that when the male penetrated a woman from behind or the side, she achieved a better orgasm than in the missionary position, and it is worth trying different positions until you find one that suits you best.

Female menopause

The menopause is a natural phase in a woman's life when her fertility draws to a close. It usually occurs between the ages of 45 and 55 with an average of 51 years. Although the menopause is dated from the last period, it is a process that starts five to ten years before, when the level of the female hormone, oestrogen, starts to fall as the ovaries slowly run out of egg follicles. Loss of oestrogen means that female sex drive can fall quickly after the menopause, especially in women who are also under stress.

Many women also find that sex feels different after the menopause. Studies suggest that a third of women experience sexual difficulties around the menopause:

- 1 in 5 lose their sex drive altogether.
- 1 in 5 suffer from vaginal dryness.
- 1 in 6 develop difficulty in reaching orgasm.
- 1 in 12 suffer from painful intercourse (dyspareunia).

These are all normal responses to falling oestrogen levels.

A few women find their sex drive increases after the menopause, however, as the increased amounts of testosterone made in their adrenal glands are no longer balanced with oestrogen or progesterone.

The most noticeable physical effect of lack of oestrogen at the menopause is vaginal dryness. Lack of lubrication means it is more difficult to become aroused and sex may be painful or uncomfortable due to dryness. The clitoris may also become less sensitive, and this is probably the main cause of difficulty reaching orgasm after the menopause. In most cases, using a special water-based lubricant gel or pessaries (e.g. KY Jelly, Replens, Senselle or Sylk – *see Resources*) will help to revitalize a flagging sex life.

As the skin is an oestrogen-sensitive tissue, this also becomes less sensitive as oestrogen levels fall. One study found that six out of ten postmenopausal women noticed skin numbness so that caresses from their partner were no longer enjoyable. Not surprisingly, nine out of ten of these women found this sensory loss interfered with their enjoyment of sex.

Another relatively common problem is clitoral hood retraction due to tissues around the vagina shrinking and thinning down due to lack of oestrogen. This can expose sensitive clitoral tissues full of nerve endings that may make sexual stimulation intensely unpleasant.

Orthodox oestrogen replacement therapy, oestrogenic herbal supplements (such as those derived from red clover or soy) or eating a diet rich in oestrogenic plants will help many of these problems. Occasionally testosterone or tibolone treatment is used where little else has helped (*see Chapters 7, 8 and 9*).

Male menopause

Male testosterone levels reach their peak in the late 20s to early 30s. Testosterone levels slowly fall after middle age, and some men develop symptoms of tiredness, irritability, a lowering of libido and a decrease in sexual performance plus excessive sweating, hot flushes and mood swings. These symptoms are similar to those occurring at the female menopause and have been referred to as the male menopause (andropause or viripause). Unlike the female menopause however, men do not experience a sudden drop in hormones. Their testosterone levels only fall slowly, by less than 1% a year beginning around the age of 40. Research suggests that abnormally low levels of testosterone are only found in 7% of men aged 40 to 60 years, 20% of men aged 60 to 80 years and around 35% of men aged over

80 years. Factors linked with an increased risk of low testosterone levels in men include heredity, obesity, stress, depression, smoking, some drugs and diet. When symptoms – including low sex drive – occur despite a normal testosterone level, this may be due to reduced interaction between circulating testosterone and its receptors (testosterone resistance), or to more testosterone becoming bound to protein (and therefore less active) in the circulation. Testosterone replacement therapy or treatment with DHEA may help (*see Chapter 8*).

Non-hormonal ways of beating the male menopause include:

- Stopping smoking.
- Drinking less alcohol.
- Taking a multi vitamin supplement as deficiencies of vitamins and minerals can exacerbate hormonal imbalances.
- Taking more exercise.
- Checking that symptoms aren't due to prescribed medications.
- Seeking counselling for relationship or sexual difficulties.

Prostate problems

The prostate is a male gland the size and shape of a large chestnut. It lies just beneath the bladder, wrapped around the urethra – the tube through which urine flows from the bladder to the outside world. After the age of 45, the number of cells in the prostate often increases and the gland starts to enlarge. This is known as benign prostatic hyperplasia or BPH for short. Prostate enlargement squeezes the urethral passage to interfere with urinary flow and causes symptoms such as:

- straining or difficulty when starting to pass water
- a weak urinary stream which may start and stop mid-flow
- passing water more often than normal, especially at night
- having to rush to the toilet
- dribbling of urine or even urinary incontinence
- discomfort when passing water
- a feeling of not emptying the bladder fully.

Half of all 60-year-old men are affected and by the age of 80, four out of five men have evidence of BPH. The exact cause is unknown, but it is thought to be linked with the action of a prostate enzyme, 5-alpha reductase, which converts the male hormone, testosterone, to a more powerful hormone, dihydrotestosterone (DHT) in the prostate gland itself. DHT seems to trigger division of prostate cells so their numbers increase.

A MORI poll of 800 males aged over 50 conducted on behalf of ProstaBrit found that almost half of sexually active males with symptoms of benign prostate enlargement had experienced a lowered sex drive, difficulty in sustaining an erection and ejaculatory problems. As a result:

- 23% of men living with a partner no longer had sex.
- 45% of sexually active men with prostate symptoms admitted to a sexual problem during the previous 12 months.
- 36% of sexually active males found sex unrewarding compared with ten years earlier.
- Men with two or more symptoms of prostate disease were more likely to wish they could have sex more often.
- Only 20% of men with prostate problems had sex at least once a month compared with 40% of men without symptoms.

A link between prostate enlargement and lowered libido was recently confirmed by an international study in which over 50% of men with BPH admitted to sexual problems, especially low sex drive. This impairment was particularly distressing for them as 72% rated sexual activity as having previously been an important part of their lives.

Sex drive in men with BPH is partly lowered as a result of anxiety about their condition, and also as a result of discomfort and the physical presence of constriction at the base of the penis. Side effects of drugs taken to help shrink the enlarged gland are also a major factor as these may affect testosterone hormone and its metabolism.

By taking natural herbal supplements to improve prostate health (e.g. zinc, saw palmetto, evening primrose oil, beta-sitosterol, rye pollen extracts) men can help to avoid prostate problems and improve symptoms that may already be present.

Hypogonadism

Underactive testicles – known as male hypogonadism – affect around 1 in 200 men. The causes are many and include pituitary under-activity, high prolactin levels (*see below*), abnormal development of the testicles including bilateral undescended testes, chromosome abnormalities, enzyme defects, surgery (e.g. castration, bilateral hernia repair with reduce blood flow to the testes), testicular disease, chemotherapy, radiotherapy, kidney failure, cirrhosis of the liver, excessive alcohol intake, sickle cell anaemia and androgen receptor deficiency. Male hypogonadism results in low sex drive and fertility problems. It may also produce symptoms of a male menopause. Once diagnosed, treatment (e.g. with testosterone replacement therapy if indicated) will usually correct low libido.

Female hypogonadism occurs naturally at the menopause when the ovaries stop working. It can occur prematurely however, or be congenital as a result of abnormal development of the ovaries, or hormone imbalances. Hormone replacement therapy, if indicated, will usually help to improve an associated low sex drive.

Prolactinoma

Raised levels of prolactin occur in 70% of patients with a benign tumour (chromophobe adenoma or prolactinoma) of the pituitary gland. The first symptom is often a total loss of sex drive, although unexpected milk production from the breasts (male and female) occasionally occurs as well. It is estimated that between 3% and 8% of men with low sex drive and impotence have raised levels of pro- lactin. It is therefore important to get your levels checked if low sex drive continues for more than three months. If diagnosed, this can be treated with a drug such as bromocriptine (*see Chapter 14*), which decreases prolactin secretion. Sometimes surgery is required as well.

Chronic disease

Many long-term diseases such as those affecting the heart, circula- tion, kidneys, liver, reproductive, urinary and nervous systems are accompanied with loss of sex drive. In some cases this is due to an imbalance of body salts, with extreme tiredness, or with physical disabilities that may cause pain, embarrassment or feelings of sexual unattractiveness. The treatment of the disease itself (e.g. certain cancers) may also have a profound effect on hormone balance, anatomy or sexuality. If your low sex drive is linked with a chronic disease, it is important to know that many other people with the same illness as yourself will have experienced similar problems. It is therefore worth contacting any relevant self-help groups dedicated to your particular type of illness to see if they can help. Often, patient self-help groups have written booklets on sexual problems or can offer advice on ways to overcome them (*see Resources*).

Relationship problems

Low sex drive can result from relationship problems, where someone has simply fallen out of love with their partner and no longer
finds them sexually attractive. Unresolved anger can also play an
important role, especially where the couple find it difficult to com-
municate. There may also be unresolved issues regarding sexual ori-
entation. Serious relationship difficulties should always be addressed
with sexual or relationship therapy such as that offered by Relate,
if the couple want to stay together. Sometimes splitting up is
inevitable, and counselling can help make separation amicable and
easier to accept without undue guilt.

Previous sexual abuse

Some women (and occasionally men) with low sex drive find sex
unpleasant or even abhorrent as a result of previous sexual abuse
or rape. Low sex drive due to these traumatic experiences should
always be helped professionally with proper counselling and psychological support.

Lack of sunshine

Lack of sunshine seems to have a damping effect on sex drive. A
young man's fancy is traditionally said to turn to love in spring (Ten-
nyson), and there is a lot of truth in this. Sunlight has an effect on the
pineal gland in the brain to promote desire and the readiness to
mate. This may explain why races with the reputation for greatest
passion tend to live in the sunniest climes. Sensible exposure to sunshine (using skin protection creams and covering up with loose, light
clothing) may therefore be beneficial for your love life.

Cultural influences

Cultural attitudes to sex vary around the world and can have a profound effect on your sex drive. In homes where sex is frowned on, parents are discreet about their sexual activity or never discuss sex, or where there is a non-sexually active, single parent raising a child, low libido becomes the normal role model. This can have a subliminal effect on a child's own sexual activity in later life – especially when they become a parent themselves.

Luckily, most cases of low sex drive can be helped by dietary and lifestyle changes, aromatherapy, homeopathy and by taking prosexual, herbal supplements.

4

Overcoming erectile problems

For a male to enjoy a normal sex life, he must have:

- an active sex drive
- the ability to achieve and sustain an erection
- the ability to ejaculate and experience a normal orgasm.

A low sex drive can result from the inability to maintain an erection, ejaculate or enjoy orgasm. Assuming that testosterone levels are normal, overcoming impotence and restoring the ability to maintain an erection and ejaculate is often accompanied by a resurgence of libido.

The structure of the penis

The bulk of the penis is formed by three cylinders of spongy tissue that run along its length and are responsible for erections. Two upper cylinders, known as the corpora cavernosa form a pair. The lower cylinder, the corpus spongiosum, runs centrally up the underside of the penis and surrounds the urinary tube (urethra). These three cylinders have an internal structure that resembles a sponge, and are divided into a series of blood-filled spaces surrounded by small blood vessels, smooth muscle fibres and elastic tissues. The three cylinders are bound together by a tough, outer fibrous sheath known as the tunica albuginea.

How erections work

For normal erection to occur the nerve and blood supply to the penis must be intact. When an erection is triggered by physical or psychological stimulation, the smooth muscle fibres in the penis relax so the blood-filled spaces become larger and arteries supplying the erectile tissues dilate. This results in a massive six-fold increase in blood flow into the penis. The spongy tissues of the penis rapidly expand and press hard against the fibrous tunica albuginea, which compresses the drainage veins running just beneath it. As a result, blood remains trapped in the engorged penis which contains up to eight times more blood than when it is flaccid.

Maintenance of erection depends upon an equilibrium between arterial blood flowing into the organ, and venous blood trickling away. Typical angles of erection at different ages are:

Age 20	110 degrees
Age 30	100 degrees
Age 40	91 degrees
Age 50	89 degrees
Age 60	75 degrees
Age 70	65 degrees

With increased age, the erection becomes less engorged due to infiltration of the spongy tissue with connective tissues, and hardening and furring up of the arteries.

For detumescence to occur, smooth muscle fibres in the spongy tissue and in the wall of the arteries contract to reduce blood flow into the organ and decrease the volume of blood that can be stored in the spongy tissues. This in turn relieves the compression on the draining veins and blood flow away from the organ rapidly increases so that flaccidity returns.

Impotence

Impotence is more properly known as erectile dysfunction. It is defined as the persistent failure to develop erections that are firm enough for satisfactory sexual intercourse.

Impotence is surprisingly common, with an estimated 1 in every 10 men affected. It becomes increasingly common with advancing age, so that 40% of men aged 40 and almost 70% of those aged 70 years are estimated to have some form of erectile dysfunction.

Of all cases of impotence, 80% have an underlying physical cause. The most common physical causes of impotence include:

- Diabetes – which can affect both the local circulation and nerve supply to the penis.
- Hardening and furring up of the arteries (atherosclerosis).
- Prescription drugs: especially those used to treat high blood pressure, depression, heart disease, gastric ulcers and cancer).
- Drugs of abuse: Long-term abuse of alcohol or drugs such as marijuana, codeine, amphetamines and heroin can cause impotence. Smoking indirectly causes impotence by increasing the effects of other risk factors such as high blood pressure and atherosclerosis.
- Leaky veins in the penis.
- Hormone imbalances.
- Previous surgery that may have affected local blood circulation or nerve supply.
- Spinal cord injury.
- Some nervous system diseases such as multiple sclerosis, Parkinsonism, Alzheimer's disease and epilepsy.

Psychological causes of impotence only account for one in five cases, and may be linked with depression, low levels of dominance and either expressed or suppressed anger. More commonly, psychological problems follow on as a result of the emotional stress of having impotence due to a physical cause. Over 20% of sufferers blamed erectile dysfunction for the break up of their relationships.

Treatment

Fortunately, more than nine out of ten men with impotence are able to regain potency with one of the many treatments now available. Treatments fall into four main groups:

- Drug Therapy
- Mechanical Aids
- Vascular Surgery
- Psychosexual Counselling

Drug therapy

A number of drugs are able to dilate blood vessels in the penis and encourage erection. These include:

- Alprostadil: injection or urethral pellet (MUSE)
- Papaverine: injection
- Phentolamine: injection
- Thymoxamine (or Moxisylyte)* injection
- Sildenafil (Viagra): oral tablet.

Until recently, the only effective way of giving drugs to treat impotence was through an injection directly into the shaft of the penis. As the drug is given into the cylinders of spongy tissue called the corpora cavernosa, this is known as intracavernosal injection. Although injections are successful in some men, others find the procedure difficult, distasteful and often painful. As a result, around one in three

---

* Now withdrawn in some countries for commercial reasons.

men stop using these injections within six months. Complications can also occur such as bleeding, formation of scar tissue (fibrosis), prolonged erections (priapism) and penile pain.

MUSE – which stands for Medicated Urethral System for Erection – is an exciting new way of delivering alprostadil into the penis without having to inject it. A special delivery device allows a pellet to be inserted painlessly into the opening of the urinary tube (urethra) at the tip of the penis. Alprostadil works by dilating blood vessels in the penis so more blood flows into the area. Erection usually follows within five to ten minutes and lasts from 30 – 60 minutes. It is associated with a low level of side effects and in a large trial, 88% of patients rated MUSE as very comfortable, comfortable or neutral to use. Most patients find MUSE preferable to intracavernosal injection.

Viagra

Viagra (Sildenafil) is another exciting advance in the treatment of impotence. It is available in some countries such as the US and the UK, and awaiting a product licence for marketing in others.

Viagra is a unique chemical belonging to a new class of drug, and is a selective inhibitor of an enzyme, Type 5 phosphodiesterase (PDE5). Viagra is thought to stimulate erection by stopping the breakdown of a chemical (cyclic GMP) involved in relaxing smooth muscle fibres in the spongy tissues of the penis (corpora cavernosa) and in the arteries supplying blood to the area. This allows more blood to flow into the penis and more to pool in the spongy tissues inside, resulting in an impressive erection once sexual stimulation starts.

Viagra is ideally taken approximately an hour before sexual activity is planned, and has been found helpful in treating impotence linked with both physical and psychological causes. In a double-blind, randomized, placebo-controlled, cross-over trial*, 92% of men

---

* All patients receive each individual treatment at some stage and all results are compared.

with impotence (aged 34 – 70 years) reported an improvement in the quality of their erections, compared with only 27% of those taking inactive placebo. This effect was independently confirmed by the men's partners. Other trials confirm a high success rate of at least 70%. The treatment is well tolerated and the most common side effects reported in various trials include headache, nasal congestion, indigestion, flushing and pelvic muscle pain. There have been reports of users suffering from heart attacks, but this may be related to the profile of those needing Viagra. Men taking it are more likely to be unfit, middle-aged or elderly males with conditions such as diabetes, high blood pressure or hardening and furring up of the arteries which caused their impotence in the first place. Possible long-term effects of treatment are not yet known, however. Viagra should not be taken by those on certain medications, such as those for treating high blood pressure or angina.

Despite the hype, Viagra will not turn normal men into sexual dynamos nor allow men to take part in feats of sexual endurance. It is a treatment for male impotence and is not an aphrodisiac. Viagra is designed to improve sexual function in men with erectile dysfunction. There is little evidence, as yet, of a direct effect on libido. Having said that, if you are suddenly able to sustain an erection after a period of impotence, you are obviously going to want to use it, and this may have a secondary effect to increase sex drive in men suffering from impotence.

Small trials are underway to see what effect – if any – Viagra may have in women. It is possible that increased blood flow to the clitoris and engorgement of the vagina may enhance sexual arousal and desire by increasing lubrication, tingling sensations and an urge to be penetrated.

Other drug treatments

Men whose impotence is associated with low levels of testosterone may benefit from testosterone hormone replacement therapy (tablets, capsules, patches, implants or injections), while men with raised levels of prolactin hormone may be helped by a drug (bromocriptine) that brings these levels down (*see Chapters 8 and 14*).

A topical cream (containing nitroglycerine) is also under trial, as is one containing aminophylline, isosorbide dinitrate and co-der-gocrine mesylate. These creams both work by dilating local blood vessels to enhance local circulation and erectile function. It is also claimed that a few drops will enhance clitoral arousal.

Yohimbine hydrochloride, derived from a tree (*Pausinystalia yohimbe* or *Corynanthe yohimbe*) native to West Africa, is available on prescription in some countries to treat male impotence at doses of around 5mg to 42mg daily (*see Chapter 9 for further information*).

Mechanical aids

Two types of mechanical aid can help impotence:

- vacuum devices
- penile implants

A vacuum device involves placing the lubricated penis in a cylinder and using a pump to create a negative pressure. This allows blood to pool in the penis and, when erection has occurred, the blood is trapped by placing an elastic ring around the base of the penis before removing the vacuum pump. The ring must be removed within 30 minutes. The penis is only rigid beyond the ring, which gives an artificial erection that has been described as cold and life-less. Some men find the device difficult or uncomfortable to use, and the ring can cause discomfort, especially during ejaculation. Some men have found it impossible to ejaculate with the ring in place.

Penile prostheses are mechanical devices designed for permanent surgical implantation into the penis to produce an artificial erection. Implants are of two main types:

- Semi-rigid rods producing half an erection all the time; they may have an embedded silver wire so they can be bent and parked when not in use, or may have a system of interlocking discs that can be rotated in one direction to lock and become rigid, and rotated the other way to disengage and become flaccid.
- Complicated inflatable devices with a small pump that is implanted in the scrotum. A fluid reservoir bag is implanted in the abdomen or pelvis and, on activation, fluid is pumped into the penile segment. Deflation depends on pressing another button so that fluid is pumped in the opposite direction.

Penile implants require open operation but can be very successful. Unfortunately, they have a relatively high failure rate requiring re-operation.

Vascular surgery

Vascular surgery can help to bypass blockages in arterial blood flow to the penis, or correct leaking veins that allow too much blood to drain away from the penis during erection.

Psychosexual counselling

Psychological or emotional factors are only responsible for one in five cases of impotence. When physical causes have been ruled out, psychotherapy or behavioural therapy can help some men and their partners. It may also help to reduce anxiety and stress in men whose impotence results from another, physical, cause (*see Chapter 13*).

Premature ejaculation

Premature ejaculation is probably the most common type of male sexual dysfunction and affects most men at some time during their life. It is usually defined as ejaculation that occurs before, or within a minute after, penetration. Premature ejaculation is particularly common amongst teenagers and tends to become less of a problem for men in their 20s and 30s and beyond. One in five men in their 20s to 30s reach orgasm within a minute of starting to make love – 62% within five minutes. Sex drive recovers quickly, usually within five to ten minutes of orgasm, however. Premature ejaculation is usually due to anxiety – especially if a new partner is involved. Ways of helping to overcome the problem include:

- Wearing a condom to reduce sensations.
- Using a local anaesthetic cream to numb the glans penis.
- Advising the male to tense his buttocks while thrusting to block nerve signals from the penis.
- Thinking of something other than sex to help damp down arousal.
- Gently pulling the testicles back down into the scrotum when they rise up to the base of the penis just before ejaculation – be careful not to twist them however.
- Using the squeeze technique – in which you squeeze the penis between thumb and two fingers just below the helmet, where the glans joins the shaft. Squeeze firmly for five seconds, then wait for a minute before resuming sex. This technique can be repeated as often as you wish.
- After experiencing premature ejaculation, successful intercourse can often occur around an hour later.
- Psychosexual Counselling.

Retarded ejaculation

Retarded ejaculation is the inability of a man to ejaculate, despite having prolonged intercourse, adequate stimulation, and an intense desire to do so. This is usually associated with tiredness, stress and distraction. It may also be linked with medical conditions such as diabetes, prostate enlargement, previous prostate surgery and some medications (eg thioridazine, antidepressants, antihypertensives).

Retarded ejaculation may be helped by ensuring surroundings are compatible with unstressful sex – quiet, warm and comfortable with no risk of interruption or being overheard. Avoid overwork, stimulants such as caffeine, smoking cigarettes and avoid alcohol. If problems persist, psychosexual counselling may be needed.

The amino acid, L-histidine, may prove helpful (*see page 60*).

5

Boosting your sex drive with pheromones

The word pheromone is derived from the Greek, *pherein* (to bring or transfer to) and *hormon* (to excite). The term literally means to bring or give excitement and these chemicals appear to live up to their name. Pheromones are volatile substances that are produced by one individual to produce powerful sexual or behavioural responses in other members of the same species. They are usually odourless and cannot be detected by the nose, but do have a profound effect on the brain.

Pheromones are well known in the animal kingdom and have been isolated from fungi, algae, barnacles, ants, termites, grasshoppers, moths and butterflies, salmon, sharks, lizards and many mammals, including mice and pigs. Interestingly, they are so far unknown in birds.

Pheromones produce powerful responses in only tiny amounts. A female gypsy moth, for example, can attract a male from several miles downwind by releasing small quantities of a sex pheromone known as gyptol. Over a six hour period, she may attract over 100 potential mates. Similarly, the female silkworm moth carries enough sex pheromone (bombykol) to work more than a billion (1,000,000,000) male silkworm moths into a frenzy. The males have special olfactory receptors on their antennae to detect the bombykol

43

scent, but the females lack receptors and are therefore unaware of their own attractiveness.

In mice and rabbits, pheromones are used to boost fertility as the female only ovulates when she detects certain pheromones excreted by males in their urine. Once fertilization has occurred, the pregnancy can be stopped if a new male is presented to a recently mated female – his pheromones cause implantation to fail, so he has the chance of impregnating her instead. Some researchers investigating the length of the human menstrual cycle when women are exposed to male odours have suggested that a similar effect may occur in humans.

It has been suspected for years that pheromones play a role in human sexual behaviour. A woman's sensitivity to musk-like odours is greatest around the time of ovulation, which some researchers interpret as proof of the ancestral presence of musky pheromones. As a result, many expensive perfumes have included secretions from the sexual glands of the musk deer, the anal glands of the civet cat and ambergris from the intestines of the sperm whale. The existence of human pheromones has only recently been confirmed, however.

The first human pheromone was isolated from skin fragments within a discarded orthopaedic plaster cast over 10 years ago. When liquid concentrates were tested on 40 volunteers they developed feelings described as a contented high with a friendly, responsive mood. Human vaginal secretions were also found to contain fatty acids identical to several thought to act as sex pheromones in other primates.

Human secretions thought to contain pheromones were then studied in the laboratory. Basically, the underarm drippings of healthy, sexually-active males and females were collected using pads worn in the armpits. After removing bacteria, odour and sweat, an alcohol fixative was added and the resulting male and female essences were studied to see if they contained any pheromone activity. In one trial, fresh male pheromones were dabbed on the upper lip of seven women with irregular menstrual cycles of 26 to 33 days.

After three months, the average length of the cycles began to approach 29.5 days – the optimum cycle length associated with highest fertility. The researchers concluded that the male essence contained at least one pheromone that helped to promote reproductive health.

The female essence was then studied in a trial in a double-blind, placebo-controlled trial, in which some women had plain alcohol dabbed under the nose rather than the active female pheromone concentrate. They found that when exposed to the sweat of other women in this way, the recipients' menstrual cycles started to synchronize with those of the women who had donated the sweat. Those exposed to inactive alcohol swabs showed no such changes. The researchers concluded that the female essence contained at least one pheromone that helped to regulate sexual function in humans. Initially, it was not known whether this effect occurred through inhalation of the odourless compounds, or by absorption through the skin. It is now thought that we may have a pheromone-detection apparatus – the vomeronasal organ, made up of chemically sensitive nerve endings – in the roof of the mouth, similar to that found in amphibians, lizards, snakes and some lower mammals. Nerve fibres from this organ are thought to lead directly to the accessory olfactory lobe of the brain, from where information is relayed to other parts of the central nervous system involved in sexual behaviour.

Human pheromones are now known to be secreted in small amounts in skin oils around the nipples, under the armpits and in the genital area. They are related to DHEA (*see page 88*), and act at a primitive, subconscious level to attract the opposite sex. Evolution has designed us to secrete pheromones when we see someone we find attractive, and when we are sexually aroused. The recipient who picks up the scent then starts releasing a few pheromones of their own. Pheromones are therefore an important key to human sexual attraction and, although they are mostly undetectable at a conscious level, have powerful effects on mood. When researchers hid male pheromones under certain chairs in a classroom, the women tended to gather around the chairs with the hidden male pheromones. Similarly, when a number of theatre programmes were sprayed with male pheromones and left on empty chairs along with unsprayed programmes, more women took the sprayed papers with them after the show than took the unsprayed ones.

Researchers studying the affect of men on the menstrual cycle of women found that in a study of women with irregular cycles, the cycles of those who lived with a man and had sex with a man once a week were more likely to be regular than those who did not. Researchers attributed the regulation to a component of male sweat. Similarly, women exposed to another woman's pheromones start to menstruate at the same time after a few months, confirming a long-noted phenomenon that women living together in institutions often develop synchronous menstrual cycles.

Even more impressively, when pheromones of women who had sexual intercourse regularly, at least once a week, were applied to women who had sex less frequently, they caused the latter to have sexual intercourse more regularly.

Many companies added animal pheromones to perfumes and aftershaves in the past to help make the wearer more sexually attractive. Exact chemical copies of human pheromones secreted by sexually attractive 25-year-old men and women are now available by mail order to add to your own favourite scent (see Resources).

These nature-identical pheromones are sexual attractants, not aphrodisiacs. They work by increasing the wearer's attractiveness to the opposite sex and to attract warmer, more intimate behaviour as a result, rather than increasing sex drive per se. In a double-blind, placebo-controlled trial, men using the active pheromone enjoyed significantly increased sexual activity and attractiveness to the opposite sex compared to those using the inactive placebo. They were found to indulge in significantly more hugging, kissing, petting and sex than before the study.

- 74% of men using the pheromone reported increased romantic attention from women.
- 47% of male users reported having sex more often than before, compared with only 9.5% of men wearing placebo.
- 41% of users kissed and petted more often than before the study, compared with only 14% of placebo users.
- 35% slept with a romantic partner more frequently than before the study, compared with only 5% of those using placebo.
- 35% of pheromone users went out on dates more often.

Women users of the female pheromone may not increase the number of times they have sex, but are more likely to have regular sex and to have regular periods. Women users have also reported that men are more attentive, courteous and pleasant, while husbands tend to become more playful, affectionate and cuddly.

Although pheromones are not classed as aphrodisiacs, you can, however, cheat, and use the pheromone intended for use by the opposite sex under your own nose to increase your own interest in sex.

These pheromones are available in liquid form and can be used by males or females to increase their own sexual interest, or to make them more attractive to the opposite sex. They pheromones may be added to perfumes or aftershaves, and are also available impregnated into candle wax for a more highly charged romantic atmosphere.

Although using bottled pheromones will help, the most subtle attractants are those produced individually by each male or female, as the message they give is then more personal. It is possible, for example, that pheromone receptors work on the lock-and-key principle so they don't send out a general message of availability but deliver coded signals to attract a specific type of partner and push away others. Researchers have analysed the way females respond to different male odours, for example, and discovered that women usually prefer men whose immune genes are *different* from their own. This is thought to help maintain the diversity of the gene pool. This changes in women taking the oral contraceptive pill however, who are more likely to prefer the smell of a man whose immune system is *similar* to their own. Researchers believe this is because hormones circulating in women on the Pill resemble those found in pregnancy – a time when women may benefit from associating with men with similar genes as they are likely to be close relatives (fathers, brothers, uncles) who will look after and protect them while they are especially vulnerable. This may give rise to problems if a woman chooses a mate while on the Pill however, and then comes off it. She may find herself wondering what she ever smelled in the whiffy guy lying next to her! Using sensual aromatherapy oils may help to overcome this problem (*see Chapter 11*).

How to use synthetic pheromones

The alcohol base of synthetic pheromones means it will evaporate if used directly on the skin. It must therefore be added to 60ml – 120ml (two to four ounces) of your favourite perfume or cologne. Adding the pheromone solution does not affect the odour of the scent it is added to. Do not add to an atomized bottle of aftershave/perfume, however, as the spray dilutes its effect.

Women: If your sex drive is low, dab a male sex pheromone under your nose or add it to your partner's aftershave. If your sex drive is fine, but your man's could do with a boost, add a female sex pheromone to your own favourite perfume.

Men: If your sex drive is low, dab a female sex pheromone under your nose or add it to your partner's perfume. If your sex drive is fine, but your female partner's could do with a boost, add a male sex pheromone to your own favourite aftershave.

You may also want to stop using antiperspirants and deodorants for a while, as these are believed to block pheromone action.

Use the pheromone-boosted scent at least every other day and wear it for at least six hours before washing it off.

The pheromones will promote sexual attractiveness and, if you wear the pheromone designed for the opposite sex, may help to boost a low sex drive – even where this is due to hormone changes, hysterectomy or advancing years. Clinicians report that 70% of women using pheromones participate in increased sexual activity compared with those not using pheromones.

Some people notice an effect within days, while for other wearers it may take up to 6 weeks to produce a noticeable response. Three out of four people respond to pheromones within two to three weeks. Interestingly, the male and female pheromones seem to act over different distances. Whereas the female pheromone can diffuse throughout a large room, the male pheromone seems to require close-up contact.

6

Boosting your sex drive with dietary supplements

A healthy sex drive depends on following a good diet and obtaining an optimum intake of vitamins and minerals. These micronutrients play a key role in reproduction and maintaining an active libido. Taking a good vitamin and mineral supplement providing around 100% of the recommended daily amount (RDA) for as many vitamins, minerals and trace elements as possible is an important part of any programme to help boost a flagging sex drive. This is especially important where low libido is linked with stress, physical tiredness, mental exhaustion, ill health, smoking or excess intake of alcohol. The following table shows why certain vitamins and minerals are important for sex drive, and good food sources.

Micronutrient (Adult EC RDA – where set)	Sexual Function	Food Sources
Vitamin A (800mcg)	Regulates sexual growth, development and reproduction by switching on genes in response to sex hormone triggers. Essential for the production of sex hormones, including oestrogen and testosterone.	Animal and fish livers, kidneys, eggs, milk, cheese, yoghurt, butter, oily fish, meat, margarine. As betacarotene: Dark green leafy vegetables and yellow-orange fruits.
B group vitamins B_1 (1.4mg) B_2 (1.6mg) B_3 (18mg) B_5 (6mg) B_6 (2mg) B_{12} (1mcg) Folate (200mcg)	Play a crucial role in energy production.	Yeast extracts, brown rice, wholegrain bread and cereals, seafood, poultry and meat (especially offal), pulses, nuts, eggs, dairy products, green leafy vegetables.
Vitamin B_6	Regulates sex hormone function and decreases production of prolactin (a hormone that reduced sex drive). In men, vitamin B_6 helps to regulate testosterone levels.	

Vitamin B$_3$ (niacin)	A fast-acting aphrodisiac in pure form and produces a flush (niacin flush) similar to the sexual flush. Enhances penile circulation by dilating blood vessels in the extremities and preventing abnormal platelet clumping. Stimulates secretion of histamine, which is needed for orgasm so intensifying the sensation.	
Vitamin C (60mg)	Essential for healthy non-clumping sperm; supplements increase semen volume and boost sex drive.	Citrus fruits, blackcurrants, guavas, kiwi fruit, green peppers, strawberries, green sprouting vegetables
Vitamin E (10mg)	Plays a key role in the manufacture of sex hormones and protects them from oxidation and degradation – deficiency is linked with a lowered sex drive and reduced fertility. May help to prevent prostatitis.	Oily fish, fortified margarine and dairy products, liver, eggs.

Boron	Needed for production of sex hormones. After just 8 days supplementation with boron, blood levels of the active form of oestrogen and testosterone double to boost sex drive in post-menopausal women.	Fruit and vegetables.
Calcium (800mg)	Plays a crucial role in muscle contraction during orgasm. May be involved in pheromone detection.	Milk, yoghurt, cheese, green vegetables, oranges, bread.
Chromium	Deficiency is linked with lowered sex drive and decreased sperm count.	Wholegrain cereals, black pepper, thyme, meat, cheese, yeast.
Copper (1.1mg)	Deficiency is linked with lowered sex drive, decreased sperm count and impotence.	Shellfish & crustaceans, yeast, olives, nuts, pulses, wholegrains, green vegetables.
Iodine (150mcg)	Deficiency produces fatigue and lowered sex drive.	Seafood, seaweed, iodised salt.
Iron (14mg)	Deficiency causes lack of energy, a common reason for going off sex, especially in women.	Red meat (especially offal), seafood, wheatgerm, wholemeal bread, egg yolk, green

		vegetables, prunes and other dried fruit.
Magnesium (300mg)	Deficiency is linked with sex hormone imbalances. Vital for sexual sensitivity, ejaculation and orgasm.	Soya beans, nuts, yeast, wholegrains, brown rice, seafood, meat, eggs, dairy products, bananas, green leafy vegetables.
Manganese	Deficiency is linked with lowered sex drive and decreased sperm count.	Black tea, wholegrains, nuts, seeds, fruit, eggs, green leafy vegetables, offal, shellfish, dairy products.
Molybdenum	Said to prevent impotence in older males.	Offal, wholegrains, green leafy vegetables, dairy products, pulses.
Phosphorus (800mg)	Necessary for maintaining sexual arousal and for semen production.	Dairy products, yeast, soya beans, nuts, wholegrains, eggs, poultry, meat and fish.
Potassium	Deficiency can reduce sex drive.	Fresh fruit and vegetables, low-salt substitutes.
Selenium	Essential for synthesis of prostaglandins which are the building	Brazil and other nuts, broccoli, mushrooms,

	blocks for sex hormones. Selenium deficiency is linked with lowered sex drive, decreased sperm count and impaired fertility. Supplements are said to boost sex drive, especially in males.	cabbage, radishes, onions, garlic, celery, wholegrains, yeast, seafood, offal.
Zinc (15mg)	Essential for male sexual maturity – deficiency reduces testicular function and can delay puberty. Lack also causes low sex drive, low sperm count, impaired fertility and impotence. Many men are zinc deficient as zinc is so important for male sexual health, each ejaculate contains around 5mg zinc – one third of the daily requirement.	Red meat (especially offal), seafood (especially oysters), yeast, wholegrains, pulses, eggs, cheese.

One of the earliest symptoms of zinc deficiency is loss of taste sensation. This can be tested for by obtaining a solution of zinc sulphate (5mg/5ml) from a chemist. Swirl a teaspoonful in your mouth. If the solution seems tasteless, zinc deficiency is likely. If the solution tastes furry, of minerals or slightly sweet, zinc levels are borderline. If it tastes strongly unpleasant, zinc levels are normal.

Vitamins and minerals for the over–50s

Those who are over 50–55 years old and have a low sex drive will need a vitamin and mineral supplement containing different doses than those needed by the under–50s. This is because with ageing, the need for most micronutrients changes due to decreased absorption from the gut and increased metabolic requirements. The only nutrients needed in lesser amounts after the age of 50 are the vitamin biotin, and the mineral iron. Those aged over 50–55 should therefore select a vitamin and mineral supplement especially designed for their age group.

Co-enzyme Q

Co-enzyme Q, also known as ubiquinone or CoQ10, is an essential, vitamin-like compound that is needed by cells to process oxygen and generate energy-rich molecules. Without CoQ10, the energy hidden in food molecules could not be converted into a form of energy that can be used by cells. It has been likened to a fuel injector in an engine that helps to concentrate fuel inside a cell so it can ignite and release energy. CoQ10 improves physical energy levels and endurance, strengthens muscles and also acts as an antioxidant.

CoQ10 is made in the liver (from the amino acid, phenylalanine) and is found in almost every food, including meat, fish, wholegrains, nuts and green vegetables. Levels of CoQ10 start to decrease over the age of 20 years however, as dietary CoQ10 is absorbed less efficiently from the intestines and its production in body cells starts to fall. Low levels of CoQ10 mean that cells do not receive all the energy they need so they function at a sub-optimal level and are more likely to become diseased, to age and even die. Studies have found that CoQ10 supplements can normalize high blood pressure, improve heart function, reduce heart disease, fight cancer and even prolong life-span.

Supplements of CoQ10 can boost energy and vitality which may have a secondary beneficial effect on sex drive.

CoQ10 is most helpful where low sex drive is linked with lack of energy, physical exhaustion, high blood pressure and coronary heart disease, as well as for those aged over 40.

Dose

Usually around 30mg – 90mg daily, with intakes of up to 180mg daily recommended for general use by some researchers. Higher doses of up to 300mg daily are used to treat illnesses such as heart disease and high blood pressure. Some studies suggest that absorption of CoQ10 is most efficient when taken as an oily solution in a soft capsule. No side effects have been reported.

It usually takes three weeks and occasionally up to three months before the full beneficial effect and extra energy levels are noticed. To utilize CoQ10 to the full, you also need to ensure a good intake of B and C vitamins.

L-arginine

L-arginine is an amino acid found in many protein foods. It increases the body's levels of an interesting nerve communication chemical (neurotransmitter) called nitric oxide (NO). NO is essential for a number of physiological processes, including increasing blood flow to the penis for normal erectile function and sexual arousal. This is in fact the way that the anti-impotence pill, Viagra works. Other actions include helping to regulate blood pressure, circulatory tone, immunity, muscle metabolism, wound healing and increased release of growth hormone.

Many researchers believe that L-arginine is one of the best all-round prosexual supplements for men. By boosting blood flow to the penis, it produces a bigger, firmer erection more frequently and may also improve sensitivity. It is helpful both for men whose sexual function is normal and for those who have erectile difficulties. In one small trial, 15 men with erectile dysfunction took placebo pills for two weeks, then took 2.8g L-arginine. None of those taking placebo noticed an effect but six noticed increased erections while receiving L-arginine although nine did not.

L-arginine is also beneficial for women as it is said to improve sexual stamina for both males and females.

Dose
150mg to 3g daily, ideally one hour before sex.
Some men require doses of 6g to achieve a noticeable effect, but this may cause an unwanted side effect of diarrhoea.

It can take two to six weeks of taking L-arginine for it to have an optimum (accumulative) effect. As it also has a short-term action however, some researchers suggest taking arginine regularly, every day, and to time the dose for about an hour before you would usually expect to have sex. L-arginine is restricted from sale in some countries.

L-arginine should not be taken by those with an autoimmune condition (e.g. rheumatoid arthritis, glomerulonephritis) except under medical supervision (studies in rats have suggested that a low arginine diet is more beneficial for immune function in these cases).

L-phenylalanine
L-phenylalanine is an essential amino acid found in many protein foods. It is involved in the synthesis of several key brain chemicals involved in regulating sex drive, such as dopamine, noradrenaline and phenylethylamine. L-phenylalanine can increase mental alertness, lift depression, boost sex drive and help to regulate appetite for food.

Usual dose (capsules, powders)

500mg – 1g per day for up to three weeks. Some nutritionists recommend taking it with B complex vitamins and high dose vitamin C for maximum effect.

Can cause stimulant side effects such as insomnia and anxiety. L-phenylalanine should not be taken if you have high blood pressure, or are taking antidepressant drugs, except under medical supervision. It should not be taken by those with a history of malignant melanoma or a metabolic condition called phenylketonuria (it may make these conditions worse).

L-tyrosine

L-tyrosine is a non-essential amino acid found in many protein foods. It can also be made in the body from another amino acid, L-phenylalanine. It is also involved in the synthesis of several key brain chemicals involved in regulating sex drive and the prosexual claims for L-tyrosine are therefore similar to those for L-phenylalanine.

Usual dose

500mg to 1g two to three times daily before meals, for up to three weeks. Some nutritionists recommend taking it with B complex vitamins and high dose vitamin C for maximum effect.

Can cause stimulant side effects such as insomnia and anxiety. L-tyrosine should not be taken if you have high blood pressure, or are taking antidepressant drugs, except under medical supervision. It should not be taken by those with a history of malignant melanoma or schizophrenia (it may make these conditions worse).

L-histidine

L-histidine is an amino acid that is converted into histamine in the body. Histamine acts as a neurotransmitter in the brain, and is the chemical that triggers orgasm when released from mast cells in the genitals and high levels of histamine therefore promote orgasm in both males and females.

Dose

50mg to 500mg twice daily with meals. No more than 1.5g daily except under medical supervision. (May be prescribed at doses of 4g daily to relieve pain in rheumatoid arthritis, for example). Some nutritionists recommend taking histamine together with B group vitamins for maximum effect.

Taking too much histamine has been linked with temporary premature ejaculation and may therefore be helpful for men with retarded ejaculation.

Histamine should not be taken by women with heavy menstrual bleeding, or anyone with a history of depression or who are taking antihistamine medications for allergic conditions.

Evening primrose oil

The beautiful evening primrose flower only blooms for a single day, but it can help your sex drive blossom year after year. Evening primrose oil (EPO) contains essential fatty acids (EFAs) needed to act as building blocks for the synthesis of sex hormones. It is estimated that 8 out of 10 people do not get all the EFAs they need from their diet.

Low sex drive is often linked with physical exhaustion and in one trial, EFA supplements showed significant beneficial effects (within three months), in 90% of people suffering from chronic fatigue. EFAs may therefore prove helpful where low sex drive is associated with lack of energy.

Evening primrose oil is a rich source of an essential fatty acid called GLA (gamma linolenic acid – sometimes shortened to gamolenic acid). The essential fatty acids are vital for the smooth functioning of the body, so much so that at one time they were collectively known as vitamin F. As they cannot be synthesized in the body, they must therefore come from the diet. There are three essential fatty acids:

- Linolenic acid (of which one type is gamma-linolenic acid).
- Linoleic acid.
- Arachidonic acid.

Linolenic acid alone is found in evening primrose oil, starflower (borage) seed oil and blackcurrant seed oil. Linoleic acid alone is found in sunflower seed, almonds, corn, sesame seed, safflower oil and extra virgin olive oil. Both linoleic and linolenic acids are found in rich quantities in walnuts, pumpkin seeds, soybeans, linseed oil, rapeseed oil and flax oil. Arachidonic acid is found in many foods (including fish, meat, dairy products and eggs) and can also be made from linoleic or linolenic acids.

Once in the body, EFAs are fed into a series of metabolic reactions (the EFA Pathway) that convert them into hormone-like substances called prostaglandins:

Linoleic acid → gamma-linolenic acid → dihomo-gamma linolenic acid (evening primrose oil) → arachidonic acid → prostaglandins

Prostaglandins are an important group of chemicals found in every body tissue. They were first discovered in the male prostate gland, hence their name.

They are involved in lots of different reactions, including control of sex drive, and sex hormone balance. You can see from the EFA pathway that some gamma-linolenic acid can be synthesized from dietary linoleic acid, but this reaction needs an enzyme (delta–6-desaturase) that is easily blocked by a number of factors, including:

- eating too much saturated (animal) fat
- eating too much trans-fatty acids (e.g. found in margarines)
- eating too much sugar
- drinking too much alcohol
- deficiency of vitamins and minerals, especially vitamin B_6, zinc and magnesium
- increasing age
- crash dieting
- smoking cigarettes
- exposure to pollution.

Many of the above factors are also linked with a lowered sex drive. When you do not get enough essential fatty acids from your diet, the metabolism can make do with the next best fatty acids available (e.g. derived from saturated fats) but as a result prostaglandin imbalances are common. Prostaglandins made from other sorts of fat cannot be converted into prostaglandins made from the EFAs. This increases the risk of sex hormonal imbalances and sexual malfunctioning.

By overcoming any enzyme blocks and feeding into the EFA pathway, food supplements containing GLA (e.g. evening primrose oil) can help to correct prostaglandin and sex hormone imbalances. As well as helping to boost a lowered sex drive, this can also damp down problems such as cyclical breast pain and chronic inflammatory diseases (e.g. rheumatoid arthritis, psoriasis and eczema). It is so effective, that in the UK, doctors can prescribe evening primrose oil to treat eczema and mastalgia (cyclical breast pain) on the NHS.

Dose
500mg – 1000mg per day for general health. To treat low sex drive linked with hormone imbalances (e.g. associated with cyclical breast

pain, premenstrual syndrome or menopausal symptoms) as much as 3g per are recommended and it can take up to three months to notice a beneficial effect.

The action of GLA is boosted by vitamin E which helps to preserve it in the body (vitamin E is a fat-soluble antioxidant). It is therefore important to take a supplement containing both GLA and vitamin E, or to take vitamin E capsules at the same time.

Certain vitamins and minerals are also needed during the metabolism of essential fatty acids. These are vitamin C, vitamin B_6, vitamin B_3 (niacin), zinc and magnesium. If you are taking evening primrose oil, you should therefore ensure that your intake of these is adequate.

Evening primrose oil supplements are safe. The only known side effect of taking too much is mild diarrhoea, though some women who have used high dose supplements for a long period of time notice that their breasts may enlarge. The only people who should not take evening primrose oil are those who are allergic to it and those with a particular nervous disorder known as temporal lobe epilepsy.

Everyone starting a prosexual programme should consider taking evening primrose oil as one of their base-line supplements.

Omega–3 fish oils

Omega–3 fish oils contain essential fatty acids (eicosapentaenoic acid) that have a beneficial effect on blood fats to reduce the risk of hardening and furring up of the arteries, heart attack, high blood pressure, stroke and erectile dysfunction linked with reduced blood circulation to the penis. Omega–3 fish oils are especially beneficial for men (or women) whose low sex drive is linked with circulatory problems that increase the risk of coronary heart disease.

Dose

Usually 1 – 4g daily. Added vitamin E stops rancidity.

Some research suggests fish oils increase blood sugar levels in diabetics. However, omega–3 fish oils protect against the increased risk of coronary heart disease that occurs in diabetes. Monitor sugar levels carefully if you are diabetic and taking fish oils. Seek medical advice before taking if you have a blood clotting disorder or are taking a blood thinning drug such as warfarin (this may increase tendency to bleed).

Royal jelly

Royal jelly (also known as bee's milk) is a milky-white substance secreted in the salivary glands of worker bees. It is a highly concentrated food given to all larvae for the first three days of their lives. After that, they're nourished on a diet of honey, pollen, and water except for the larva that is destined to become a queen bee. She will continue to be fed on royal jelly to stimulate and sustain her development. As a result, the queen bee grows 50% larger than other genetically-identical female bees (worker bees), and has a lifespan that is nearly 40 times longer.

Royal jelly is a rich source of essential amino acids, essential fatty acids, sugars, sterols and phosphorous compounds as well as acetylcholine – a neurotransmitter needed to transmit messages from one nerve cell to another. Royal jelly is also an excellent source of vitamin B_5 (pantothenic acid) and a possibly therapeutic substance called 10-hydroxydec–2-enoic acid. There is some evidence that royal jelly can decrease blood cholesterol levels and may be helpful for those whose low sex drive is linked with abnormal blood fat levels and poor circulation.

Royal jelly is traditionally taken as an energizing tonic, to prolong youthfulness and to improve the complexion. It also seems to alleviate anxiety, sleeplessness and memory loss and boosts the immune system. It is widely reputed to help rejuvenate a low sex drive. It needs to be blended with honey (or powdered in capsules) to preserve the active ingredients during storage.

Dose
50 to 100mg per day

Best kept refrigerated and taken on an empty stomach.
NB avoid if you are allergic to bee products.

Bee pollen
Bee pollen is an ultrafine dust produced on the anthers of male flowers which is composed of male sex cells. Bees collect the pollen when foraging for nectar and inadvertently transfer some to the ovaries of female flowers to fertilize them. Collected bee pollen is then stored in the hive as food for young bees. Bee pollen is a very nourishing substance, rich in amino acids, carbohydrates, fatty acids, vitamins, minerals and trace elements. In ancient Greece and Italy, bee pollen was considered a tonic food for those wanting greater energy, vibrancy, zest for life – and a healthy sex drive. Ambrosia, the secret food of the Gods that was said to guarantee eternal life, was made from a combination of honey, bee pollen and beebread (the pollen stored in the honeycomb cells).

Bee pollen is widely reputed to boost energy levels, libido, sexual potency and fertility. It is also said to reduce hot flushes in menopausal women and to alleviate male symptoms of an enlarged prostate gland.

Dose
250mg – 2g daily for at least one month.

Avoid if you are allergic to bee products or to pollen.

Blue-green algae

Blue-green algae (e.g. Chlorella, Spirulina, Aphanizomenon flos aquae) are a rich source of vitamins, minerals and amino acids that can give your sex drive a natural green energy boost.

Blue-green algae are a wholefood source of over 100 synergistic and easily assimilated nutrients including antioxidants, vitamins, minerals, enzymes, essential fatty acids, essential and non-essential amino acids, iron, chlorophyll, protein and other protective substances. Gram for gram, it is richer than any other source of natural betacarotene which protects against cell damage and ageing. It is therefore a useful supplement for those whose low sex drive is linked with tiredness, exhaustion and lack of energy.

Dose

Varies from product to product. Typically 3g daily. Large amounts may be consumed as a food without apparent harm. Some products have been contaminated with toxic algae, so ensure you take a recognized, main-stream brand – preferably one certified organic.

Choline, phosphatidyl choline and lecithin

The closely related supplements, choline, phosphatidylcholine and lecithin may be able to boost sex drive by acting as building blocks to stimulate production of certain neurotransmitters in the brain, including acetylcholine, noradrenaline and dopamine which help to regulate mood and sex drive. Phosphatidyl choline is also needed to make cell membranes, including those found in the nervous and reproductive systems.

Choline has also been shown to help improve memory and cognition.

Dose

Choline (powder, tablets, capsules, liquid): 100 to 500mg daily is usually all that is needed. Can be taken in doses as high as 1g three times a day for improving mental function.

Phosphatidylcholine (capsules): 1g to 2g daily.

Lecithin (granules, capsules, liquid): 5g to 10g.

These supplements should ideally be taken with vitamin B_5 to improve their effect in the body.

Should not be used by those with manic depression as it may make their condition worse.

Soy bean extracts

Soy beans are known as *ta tou* in Chinese, which means greater bean. Soy extracts are now widely available as a food supplement aimed at middle-aged and older women to help ease the loss of oestrogen in later life.

Soy beans are a rich source of isoflavones – plant hormones that have a similar structure to oestrogen and corticosteroid hormones produced by the adrenal glands. The principle isoflavones found in soy are: daidzein, genistein and glycitein. These phytoestrogens can bind to oestrogen receptors in the body, to give the benefits of oestrogen without the risks. The isoflavonoids in soybeans have about 0.2% of the oestrogen activity of the main human oestrogen, oestradiol. Confusingly, phytoestrogens are also beneficial in high oestrogen states, as they compete for oestrogen receptors with the stronger oestrogens, thereby having an anti-oestrogen effect. In addition, phytoestrogens may reduce the effects of oestrogens in the body by stimulating production of sex hormone binding globulin (SHBG), which binds oestrogen in the circulation to reduce its effects.

Soy is also a good source of other phytosterols that may help production of testosterone hormone. In Japan, Asia, the Mediterranean and Latin American communities the average person consumes 20 to 100mg of soy isoflavones per day and has a sex drive that is renowned. The typical western diet provides only 2 – 5mg isoflavones per day. Increasing intake of soy products is likely to have a beneficial effect on libido and will confer many other health advantages.

Soy isoflavones also have an antioxidant action and have been found to help reduce cholesterol levels, inflammation and to protect against certain diseases of the heart, kidney and gall bladder. They may help to increase muscle strength, stamina and endurance and may have an anticancer action. Some scientists believe that eating just one bowl of miso soup (made from fermented soya beans) per day may reduce the risk of stomach cancer by more than 30%, for example.

Dose
A daily intake of at least 50mg isoflavones is recommended.

NB 60g of soy protein provides 45mg isoflavones.

Chicken egg extracts
Chicken egg extracts are one of the latest supplements to be promoted as prosexual agents. They are available under the brand names of Ardor in the US, Libido in the UK, and Libid, Libbido, Erosom and Ardorare in other markets.

Egg consumption has long been associated with sexual potency. When Casanova wanted to build up his strength, he is said to have consumed large quantities of raw egg to boost his levels of testosterone. We now eat far fewer eggs than our ancestors, and perhaps more significantly do not eat farm-fresh, free-range eggs that are likely to have been fertilized. Instead we eat unfertilized, unincubated, battery-hen eggs that do not contain the prosexual hormone-like substances. It has even been suggested that this dietary change has contributed to the development of low sex drive in some people.

Chicken egg extracts (CEE) have been found to enhance sex drive in males. The exact way in which they work is not understood. After nine days incubation, the fertilized eggs have reached a critical stage of pre-embryonic development and contain a variety of high molecular weight substances which, when freeze-dried and consumed, are thought to increase the effects of testosterone in the body.

CEE has been shown to have a positive effect in several studies, involving otherwise healthy, middle-aged males complaining of a low sex drive. Within two weeks of taking CEE, 58% reported a consistently higher sexual desire compared with those taking inactive placebo. Beneficial effects were usually noticed within two weeks.

A randomized, placebo-controlled, double-blind, cross-over, clinical trial of 31 male volunteers with low sex drive was conducted in Norway. Without knowing what they were given, half the men received CEE for the first three weeks of the study, then received inactive placebo for three weeks. The other half received inactive placebo for the first three weeks, then CEE.

The men rated their sex drive daily by marking a cross on a 0 to 10cm visual analogue scale where 0cm = no change in sex drive, and 10cm equalled a very pronounced change.

During the first week in those receiving CEE first, the average sex drive rating was 0.25cm (i.e. little change in sex drive). By the third week, the men gave their sex drive an average rating of almost 8cm out of a possible 10cm (pronounced increase in sex drive). Within a week of starting placebo however, sex drive rating fell to 3cm (little change) and was back to less than 1cm (i.e. very little change in sex drive compared with before the trial started) within three weeks of starting the placebo.

In the men given placebo for the first three weeks followed by CEE for three weeks, average sex drive ratings were low (less than 1cm). After taking CEE for three weeks however, the men noticed a pronounced increase in sex drive compared with before the trial, marking a cross almost at 8cm on the scale, on average.

In a Swedish trial, 31 males with low sex drive took CEE for three weeks. Overall, 84% of men experienced a good response with an overall increase in their desire for sexual activity. Almost half (45.2%) experienced a major or very pronounced increase in sex drive. Only 16.1% of men noticed no increase in libido. No participants reported any side effects. As well as increasing sex drive, the subjects reported improved self-esteem as a result. Most wanted to continue taking the product.

US trials have shown extracts increase intensity and frequency of desire, intensity of orgasm, general wellbeing, feelings of happiness and energy levels from an average pre-treatment level of 9% to a post-treatment level of 31%.

A trial in Canada involved 18 patients who had low sex drive as a result of antidepressant therapy. A course of CEE increased their average number of sexually arousing thoughts per week from two to 15 after five weeks, and the number of times they initiated sexual activity increased from an average of one to 5.5 times per week, and the rate of successful intercourse increased three-fold from an average of 0.7 to an average of 2.2 times per week.

A large-scale study involving 1000 patients in a multi-centre double-blind clinical study is also underway in Canada and the US.

Trials are also planned to investigate the possible effect of CEE on females following beneficial effects on both men and women whose low sex drive was linked with anti-depressant medication. CEE produced a definite to very pronounced increase in sexual activity in 88% of cases. These benefits were noted within two to three weeks.

CEE would benefit any male with a low sex drive, including those whose symptoms are linked with antidepressant therapy. Many men noticed a beneficial effect after three day's treatment, with the full effect developing within three weeks.

Dose

First week: 6 capsules twice a day, morning and evening.
Thereafter: 2 capsules twice a day.

Each 450mg capsule contains 434mg active ingredients. Also available as a powdered drink containing CEE plus aniseed, ginseng, rosemary, peppermint, hops, chamomile, thyme, clove and fennel plus vitamin B_{12}, folic acid and thiamine. Dissolve one sachet in a glass of cold water or juice once a day.
CEE is 90% cholesterol free. Avoid if you are sensitive to hens' eggs.

Gamma-hydroxybutyrate

Gamma-hydroxybutyrate (GHB) is only included here for information in case you come across it and are tempted to use it. Although its possession is not against the law, its supply is illegal in some countries. GHB is a natural metabolic substance found in every cell of the body and also in animal foods. It has a powerful prosexual action, but unfortunately, there are concerns about possible serious adverse side effects from taking it in supplement form. These concerns result from the fact that GHB produces a euphoria which mimics that of many illicit drugs, and it may therefore have the potential for addiction when used regularly in high doses. As a result of these concerns, GHB is unavailable over the counter in some countries, and may also be unavailable on prescription. It is included here for completeness, however, as there is a thriving black-market in the supplement yet many people taking it are unaware of how it works or the possible dangers.

When gamma-hydroxybutyrate (GHB) reaches the brain, some of it is converted to an amino acid, gamma-aminobutyric acid (GABA). GABA acts as an inhibitory neurotransmitter which helps to regulate nerve cell activity. It is thought to induce feelings of calm and tranquillity by damping down the action of nerve cells involved in anxiety, agitation and manic behaviour.

GHB also increases brain levels of dopamine, including that found in the substantia nigra which helps to regulate sex drive (*See deprenyl/selegiline Chapter 14*). In addition, it increases production of prolactin hormone. Increased prolactin levels would usually be expected to reduce sex drive (as when breastfeeding, *see pages 21–22*) but this effect seems to be masked by the cumulative effect of the other prosexual actions of GHB.

GHB produces a state of relaxation, euphoria and disinhibition similar to that of alcohol. It also increases skin sensitivity and intensifies orgasm, although it takes longer to achieve. In males, it also enhances erections. Side effects are similar to those of alcohol, with excess leading to dizziness, giggling, slurred speech, loss of co-ordination, sleepiness and unconsciousness according to the amount taken.

Dose

Bear in mind that GHB is nicknamed GBH (Grievous Bodily Harm). Not recommended. If deciding to use it, do so only in a safe environment, with people you trust, in case you become unconscious and could be taken advantage of.

For a more positive overview and further information about GHB, read: *Better Sex Through Chemistry*, by John Morgenthaler & Dan Joy (*see Resources for details*).

7

Boosting your sex drive with food

Diet can have a profound effect on your sexuality – and not just by providing vitamins, minerals or aphrodisiacs. The food you eat undoubtedly influences your hormone balance and can affect your sex drive. As part of a prosexual programme, it is important to follow a healthy diet that is relatively low in fat, but contains beneficial fatty acids such as those found in fish, evening primrose, olive or linseed oils. Eat plenty of fresh fruit and vegetables (at least five servings per day) and eat as wide a variety of wholefoods as possible. Other important pro-sexual dietary tips include:

- Be a grazer rather than a gorger. Eat little and often during the day to keep your blood sugar levels constant – fresh or dried fruit is ideal as a snack.
- Balance your intake of saturated and polyunsaturated fats.
- Avoid or limit your intake of sugar, salt, tea, coffee and other caffeinated drinks.
- Avoid convenience, pre-processed foods and additives – eat home-made meals as much as possible.
- Reduce your salt intake by avoiding obviously salty foods and not adding salt (sodium chloride) during cooking or at the table – use herbs and black pepper for flavour and,

where salt is essential, use mineral-rich rock salt rather than table salt.

● Aim to drink plenty of fluids – preferably mineral water or herbal teas.

Going organic

Going organic is strongly recommended as part of your prosexual programme. A wide range of agro-chemicals such as pesticides, weed killers, fungicides, fumigants, growth promoters, growth retardants and fertilizers have been linked with ill health. Some affect hormone balance in the body and may well play a role in reduced sex drive, reduced sperm count and reduced fertility. These chemicals are often applied to plants regularly, from the time the crop is still in its seed form, during germination and throughout its growing cycle. Each non-organic apple, for example, has been dosed around 40 times with up to 100 additives, before you eat it. These chemicals do not just lie on the surface of the produce, but are found beneath the skin and sometimes throughout the flesh itself. While these chemicals are considered safe to use on crops, the full effects of many on our long-term health, immunity and reproductive system are still not fully understood. That's why increasing numbers of people are deciding to go organic. Apart from anything else, research shows that organic foods contain, on average, twice the nutrient content of commercially grown produce. This is partly because they contain less water and more solid matter, but is also due to the multi-rich soils in which they are grown.

Natural plant oestrogens

Many plants contain natural chemicals that have a weak, hormone-like action in the human body. These plant hormones, known as phytoestrogens and phyto-progesterones, can help to balance levels of female hormones in the body and can improve symptoms such as premenstrual syndrome, menopausal hot flushes and night sweats, fatigue and associated low sex drive. While these plant hormones are especially beneficial for middle-aged and older women, they also have positive health advantages for men and may help to reduce the risk of prostate disease, for example.

Plants rich in oestrogen-like substances include:

Seeds: almost all, especially linseeds, pumpkin seeds, sesame seeds, sunflower seeds and sprouted seeds (e.g. alfalfa, mung beans, lentils, red clover, soya beans).

Nuts: especially almonds, cashew nuts, hazelnuts, peanuts, walnuts and nut oils.

Wholegrains: almost all, especially corn, buckwheat, millet, oats, rye, wheat.

Fresh fruits: apples, avocados, bananas, mangoes, papayas, rhubarb.

Dried fruits: especially dates, figs, prunes and raisins.

Vegetables: Dark green leafy vegetables (e.g. broccoli, Pak choi, spinach, spring greens, watercress), celery, fennel and exotic members of the cruciferous family (e.g. Chinese leaves, kohl rabi).

Legumes: especially soy beans and soy products (e.g. tofu, tempeh, miso, tamari), chickpeas, lentils.

Kitchen Garden Herbs: especially angelica, chervil, chives, garlic, ginger, horseradish, nutmeg, parsley, rosemary and sage.

Honey: especially that made from wild flowers.

For information on oestrogenic herbal supplements, *see Chapter 9.*

A bread fortified with soya and linseed to make it rich in natural plant oestrogens is now also available in supermarkets (Burgen bread). Eat it for its delicious taste – any health benefits are a welcome bonus.

Aphrodisiac foods

The following foods have all gained a reputation as aphrodisiacs in the past. Oysters are renowned, for example, and may even be beneficial as a result of their high mineral zinc content. Many other supposed aphrodisiacs seem only to have gained notoriety as a result of their suggestive shape and the way they linger on the lips and nostrils. The following prosexual foods are included just for fun – incorporate them into your diet to form your own opinion on whether or not they actually work.

Aniseed

Aniseed and Star Anise are both mildly stimulating aphrodisiacs that were powdered and combined with honey to form an aphrodisiac paste. This was applied to the genitals in Ancient India for an explosive effect. Aniseed was also a principle ingredient of a rich, spicy cake served at Roman weddings to boost the sex drive of newly-weds. The essential oil content is 2 – 3% and mainly consists of anethole.

Apples

A symbol of fertility that have always been associated with love, as they were sacred to Rhianno, Celtic goddess of love and marriage.

Artichokes

Known as aphrodisiacs in France, where there is a saying: Artichokes, like wine, are good for ladies when gentlemen eat them.

Asparagus Tips

The Egyptians, Greeks, and Romans all valued asparagus as an aphrodisiac. The herbalist Culpeper also wrote that 'a decoction of asparagus roots could stirreth up bodily lust in man or woman'.

Best eaten with the fingers and dripping with butter. One drawback is the revolting odour that gives urine a smell similar to severe cystitis.

Aubergines

Aubergine (also known as eggplant or the apple of love) is regarded as an aphrodisiac in its native India. The Kama Sutra suggests rubbing your partner's body with aubergine juice to increase their libido for a month.

Bananas

Bananas are one of the few foods with real potential as an aphrodisiac – and not for their phallic shape. Bananas contain an alkaloid (bufotenine) that acts on the brain to increase mood, self-confidence and possibly increase sex drive. It is found in greatest quantity just beneath the skin, and is best obtained by cutting whole bananas lengthways and baking them with a little sugar. The flesh should then be scraped away from the skin before eating.

Basil

Basil has a reputation as a strong aphrodisiac in Mexico and Italy. Combine with pine nuts and garlic in Pesto sauce for a more racy effect. Adding a mashed, grilled tomato softens the flavour and boosts its libidinous activity.

Black pepper

Pungent black pepper has a reputation for bringing spice to the bedroom as well as the palate.

Carrot

The Ancient Greeks believed that all parts of the carrot were aphrodisiac and ate the seeds, root and foliage when preparing for an orgy.
They were known as 'philon', meaning loving and were given to
potential sex partners to stimulate their ardour.

Caviar

The salty, musky aroma and pungent flavour of caviar is a renowned
aphrodisiac that is said to remind lusty males of the female genitals.
Caviar may well contain steroidal compounds that might boost sex
drive but probably only in quantities that few people can afford.

Celery

Celery – like the truffle – is said to contain an aphrodisiac substance
similar to a pig pheromone which also has a prosexual action in
humans.

Chicory

Chicory was commonly included in medieval love potions and was
given to lovers to encourage faithfulness.

Chocolate

Eating chocolate can increase brain levels of several chemicals,
including mood-altering PEA (phenylethylamine) which produces a
mild, confidence-instilling buzz. Chocolate also contains tryptophan
– a chemical converted to serotonin in the body, and theobromine,
which peps you up – three reasons why chocolate is so addictive.
The fourth reason is that chocolate uniquely melts in the mouth at
body temperature – to produce a silky, luscious sensation that is
distinctly sexual.

Cucumbers
Cucumber probably gained its reputation as an aphrodisiac due to its suggestive length and circumference.

Durian
The prickly fruit of the durian tree (Durio zibethinus), native to Borneo, Malaya, Thailand and the Philippines is a renowned aphrodisiac. An ancient Malay saying declares that 'When the durians fall, the sarongs rise.' The spherical fruit measures 15 to 20cm in diameter and contains five oval compartments, each filled with a cream-coloured, custard-like pulp containing one to five chestnut-sized seeds. The pulp is edible, and the seeds may be eaten if roasted. The durian has a pungent odour, which has been compared to that of strong cheese, but is mild and sweet to taste. It is so prized as an aphrodisiac that owners frequently sleep under the trees as harvesting nears, to protect their crop. The fruit is seldom exported as local demand is so high.

Eggs
Eggs – especially free-range fertilized eggs – contain steroidal substances that seem to enhance libido (*see page 68*). Battery-laid eggs won't work – so go for naturally farmed quails eggs, duck eggs, barn-laid farm eggs, caviar and even snail's eggs, which are more likely to have been fertilized.

Fennel
Fennel has an ancient reputation as an aphrodisiac that stimulates the genitals of those who eat it and stimulates desire.

Fenugreek
Fenugreek seeds are considered aphrodisiac, tonic and cleansing.

Figs

The fig is considered sensual and erotic for when the fruit is slit open, the juicy, pale pink flesh is apparently reminiscent of the female genitalia. In some cultures, figs are thrown at newlyweds in place of rice.

Garlic

Garlic can improve feelings of wellbeing and boost sex drive (*see page 130*). In one study, those taking standardized garlic powder tablets for four months noticed a significant improvement in positive mood characteristics such as increased activity, happiness, ability to concentrate and sensitivity, while at the same time, negative mood characteristics such as anxiety and irritation were reduced.

Ginger

Ginger is one of the oldest medicinal spices and aphrodisiacs known. It was taken regularly by Confucius, the great philosopher of the 5th and 4th centuries BC, who helped to make it popular in China. Ginger is a warming, stimulating spice that can increase blood circulation and ginger up your sex drive.

Honey

Honey contains bee pollen which may account for its reputed pro-sexual effect. Honey was widely used in poultices applied to the lingam (male member) to increase its size in ancient India, and mixed with crocodile dung, olive oil and lemon juice for use as a contraceptive pessary by women.

Leeks

Like its close relations, garlic and onions, leeks have a long reputation as a powerful aphrodisiac.

Lobster

Lobster (and its close relative, crayfish) are considered aphrodisiacs both for their delicate, seafood taste and their expense which makes them a luxury item.

Lychee

Lychee is said to be aphrodisiac for a male, if he skins the fruit, gently extracts the stone, and then inserts the tip of his tongue in the crevice that remains.

Mango

In India, the mango is believed to boost sex drive and prolong lovemaking.

Melons

In ancient Persia, melons were considered an aphrodisiac and eaten regularly to stimulate the appetite for both food and love. Melon is still commonly served as a starter for meals in many cultures.

Mushrooms

Raw mushrooms – like truffles – have an odour reminiscent of sex and were widely regarded as aphrodisiacs by the Ancient Romans and Greeks.

Nutmeg

Nutmeg contains an amphetamine-like chemical which is harmless in small quantities. If, however, grated nutmeg is mashed with avocado flesh and chilled overnight, a chemical reaction occurs that is said to produce a prosexual effect in men.

Oats

Oats are a nutritious aphrodisiac that may be taken as porridge or in supplement form (*see page 152*).

Onions

Like their close relation, garlic, onions are reputed to be a powerful aphrodisiac and celibate ancient Egyptian priests were forbidden to eat them. Ovid advised that eating onions stirred the passions, and Onion Soup is recommended in France as a restorative to relight the fires of desire after an exhausting first wedding night.

Oysters

Oysters are probably the most famous aphrodisiac food of all time. They were especially popular in Edwardian times, for they were extremely cheap as was champagne – the drink they undoubtedly mix with best. Raw oysters owe their aphrodisiac reputations to their salty, marine odour, their plump resemblance to the female genitalia and their high zinc content.

Passion Fruit

The Passion vine is named for biblical reasons due to its complex flower structure: the five sepals alternating with five petals are said to symbolize the crucifixion, the inner corona of filaments represents the crown of thorns and the styles depict the cross and nails. Nevertheless, the passion fruit is commonly regarded as an aphrodisiac.

Peaches

The luscious, juicy peach has a shape suggestive of a young maiden's buttocks and was highly regarded in ancient China as an aphrodisiac that increases the frequency of sexual intercourse.

Peanuts

Peanuts contain histidine, an amino acid that can trigger and intensify orgasm.

Pine kernels

The Romans considered pine nuts to have powerful aphrodisiac properties. Together with basil and garlic they make Pesto sauce a gourmet dish for lovers.

Pomegranate

The pomegranate is believed by some to be the fruit that tempted Eve in the Garden of Eden, rather than the apple. The Kama Sutra recommends splitting the blushing, golden globe in two and sharing it for a night of incomparable passion and boosted fertility.

Prunes

Prunes were served in medieval brothels to promote sex drive in both customers and jaded girls.

Saffron

Saffron, the dried pistils of a crocus, is considered a powerful aphrodisiac in Spain, India and China. It is traditionally taken to maintain sexual performance in males.

Sauerkraut

According to researchers in Pittsburgh, sauerkraut has a definite pro-sexual action for males. After 450 volunteers ate three plates of German pickled cabbage a day, 90% said that jaded sexual appetites had been banished and they were able to make love every day for up to 30 minutes. They claim that sauerkraut's high content of vitamin C and lactic acid is responsible for increased sexual activity.

Sesame Seed

Sesame seeds were widely used in the Orient to promote fertility. An Arab powder made from sesame, ginger, cloves, nutmeg, coriander, cardamom and lavender was widely used as an aromatic aphrodisiac in ancient times.

Shrimps

Shrimps contain phenylalanine – an amino acid that promotes sex drive (*see page 58*) – and zinc.

Strawberries

Strawberries are known as the fruit of Venus – the Roman goddess of love. They are regarded as an aphrodisiac, especially when combined with champagne.

Tomatoes

Tomatoes originate from South America where they were first cultivated by the Aztecs. Legend has it that a 16th century Spanish priest brought tomato seeds to Seville from Peru. They had such as positive effect on those who ate them that the French referred to them as *pommes d'amour*, or apples of love.

Truffles

Truffles are the next most famous aphrodisiac food after oysters. They have an odour reminiscent of the pheromone given off by male pigs, hence are readily snuffled out by amorous sows. Both the white and black variety are said to be potent.

Vanilla

Vanilla is said to be a potent aphrodisiac, and is widely used in perfumery and aromatherapy (*see page 206*). The effects of its sensual aroma may be intensified by eating vanilla-flavoured confections.

Sexy weekend diet for two

Using the above list of aphrodisiac foods, it is easy to construct a prosexual diet for a sexy weekend for two. Although there's no guarantee it will work, you will certainly have fun eating it and trying.

Friday evening
Caviar on toast
Mushrooms Stuffed with tomatoes, basil, pine nuts and truffle
Fresh mango with vanilla sauce
Champagne

Saturday breakfast
Fresh Melon
Toast with honey

Saturday lunch
Celery and leek soup
Asparagus tips with lashings of butter and black pepper
Chocolate mousse

Saturday dinner
Half a dozen oysters
Lobster with shrimp sauce
Fresh lychees plus vanilla ice cream
Champagne

Sunday breakfast
Oaty porridge with grated nutmeg

<u>Sunday lunch</u>
Onion soup
Cucumber, fennel, celery and chicory salad
Mushroom and garlic bake
Fresh figs with strawberry and passion fruit salad

<u>Sunday dinner</u>
Carrot and ginger soup
Baked aubergine with Pesto sauce
Baked bananas
Champagne

8

Boosting your sex drive with hormones

Your sex drive depends on the level of a variety of hormones and brain chemicals (*see Chapter 2*). Their interaction is complex and imbalances can have a profound effect on your physical and emotional wellbeing, as well as adversely affecting your sex drive. Several hormones are now available – either over-the-counter or on prescription – to help boost a low libido, including:

- dehydroepiandrosterone (DHEA)
- pregnenolone
- testosterone
- androstenedione
- oestrogen
- natural progesterone
- tibolone
- human growth hormone.

Hormones are vitally important for all aspects of health, including a normal sex drive. They are chemical messengers secreted in tiny amounts directly into the blood stream. They interact with special receptors to trigger powerful responses in certain target tissues. Some hormones (e.g. adrenaline) work within seconds of their release by changing the activity of cell enzymes to speed up or slow down your metabolism. Others (e.g. oestrogen) work more slowly through a direct action on cell chromosomes. They can literally switch individual genes on or off to increase production of important proteins and enzymes, including those needed for regulating sex drive.

Low sex drive is often linked with a hormone imbalance. These imbalances may be investigated in a number of ways, including blood or saliva tests to measure levels of individual sex hormones.

Do not use any of the following hormonal supplements without medical advice – this is especially important for men with a prostate problem, or anyone with a history of a hormone sensitive condition (including some cancers). Do not use during pregnancy or when breastfeeding unless individually prescribed by a doctor for medical reasons.

Dehydroepiandrosterone (DHEA)

DHEA is a hormone made in the adrenal glands. Its main function is to act as a building block for producing other steroid hormones including the sex hormones, oestrogen, progesterone and testosterone as well as corticosteroids. For many years, this was thought to be its sole function. It is now known, however, that cells contain specific DHEA receptors, suggesting that this mother hormone may also have its own particular functions.

Most DHEA circulates in the body in the form of DHEA-sulphate (DHEA-s) as a sulphate molecule is added to DHEA when it reaches the liver. DHEA-s is generally considered to be less active than DHEA, but it is usually this level which is measured and used to give an accurate reflection of DHEA status in the body.

DHEA levels are slightly higher in men than women, and levels decline with age in both sexes. Production peaks around puberty and stays high until the late twenties, after which there is a continuous decline. At the age of 20, we naturally produce around 30mg per day; this drops to less than 6mg daily by the age of 50. This reduction in DHEA levels is believed to contribute to the increased risk of a number of age-related conditions such as diabetes, obesity, elevated cholesterol levels, heart disease, arthritis and autoimmune diseases.

DHEA has been found to increase a flagging sex drive and is also claimed to have a number of almost astonishing beneficial effects such as:

- regulating immune function to reduce the severity of infections and auto-immune disorders
- improving physical and emotional wellbeing
- decreasing body fat percentage
- regulating sugar control
- lifting a low mood
- increasing energy levels
- reducing the adverse effects of stress
- enhancing memory and mental clarity
- reducing the risk of coronary heart disease
- reducing the risk of osteoporosis
- reducing the risk of dementia
- reducing the risk of impotence
- possibly extending life span – it is becoming known as the fountain of youth.

DHEA is thought to increase sex drive by increasing circulating levels of androgens (the masculinizing hormones, androstenedione, testosterone and dihydrotestosterone) in both sexes. As its levels do not fall dramatically at the menopause it is thought by some to help sustain female sex drive as levels of oestrogen fall. Research findings regarding DHEA and sex drive are conflicting, however.

In one study, men and women aged 40 – 70 years took 50mg of DHEA nightly for three months. This was found to double levels of androgens in women, but to only produce a small rise in androstene-dione in men. Treatment was associated with a marked increase in perceived physical and psychological wellbeing for both men (67%) and women (84%) but the volunteers reported no change in libido.

In another study, DHEA was taken by 5 postmenopausal women aged 60 to 70, for one year. The DHEA was given as a 10% cream applied in the morning on the inner thighs. The dose was adjusted according to blood results to give similar levels to those found in women aged 20 and 30. After one year, 80% of the women reported increased wellbeing and 80% reported a marked increase in sex drive. There was also a significant improvement in vaginal dryness and no over-stimulation of the womb lining (endometrial hyperpla-sia). While there was no change in body weight, there was a 10% reduction in body fat which was replaced by lean muscle, and bone density increased. Some of the women developed mild acne but there were no serious side effects.

DHEA is readily available in some countries, such as the US, but is unavailable in others, such as the UK and Canada. In the US, DHEA is available over the counter and has spawned a multi-million dollar industry. Many people believe DHEA should only be available on prescription, however. Others feel that if it is used responsibly, it should remain available over-the-counter. The best approach for those who feel DHEA may be beneficial is to consult a medical doctor who will measure DHEA levels, prescribe the hormone if indicated, and provide regular follow-up monitoring (e.g. every quar-ter) to ensure normal youthful levels are achieved.

Optimal blood levels of DHEA are 750ng/dl or above for men, and 550ng/dl or above in women (test kits are available, see resources).

Dose

It is best to take DHEA under the supervision of a physician who is familiar with its potential side effects. If you are under 40, it is best to have your levels of DHEA/DHEAS determined (through either a blood or saliva test) to see if you need supplementation and, if so, to determine the right dose. DHEA requirements vary from person to person. It is important not to take too much – smaller dosages may be as effective and safer. When taking DHEA for low sex drive, it is usual to start with a low daily dose of 5 – 10mg and to increase if this is ineffective, up to a dose range of 25 – 50mg a day. Some physicians recommend smaller doses of 2 – 8mg DHEA, taken every other day or, if taken daily, to stop them for a week or two after every month of treatment.

DHEA is available in a variety of formulations: pills, capsules, sublingual tablets, cream form, tablets, liquid and even spray. New research suggests that oral hormones should be taken with food as twice as much is absorbed when digested with meals than when taken on an empty stomach.

The possible unwanted side effects of DHEA include:

- Acne and other skin rashes
- unwanted hair growth in women
- mood changes such as irritability
- over-stimulation
- increased heart rate and palpitations
- insomnia
- tiredness, fatigue and lack of energy
- possible increased risk of cancer of the breast or ovaries in women, and of prostate cancer in men
- transient hepatitis and increased pressure in the eyes have also been reported.

If used appropriately, in low doses, side effects are less likely. Excess may cause masculinization in women with the development of facial hair and a deeper voice. This is only usually seen in doses greater than 25mg a day and is most common at doses above 90mg per day. Some doctors feel women should not take DHEA at all. Others feel it is acceptable to take it over the age of 40 as long as androgen levels are being measured regularly.

Because DHEA is converted into oestrogen in the body, it may affect the dose of HRT required by those taking it.

As some DHEA is converted into oestrogen, there is a possibility of breast enlargement in men taking high doses long-term.

Although reports of serious problems are infrequent, the long-term safety of using DHEA regularly for many years is not yet known. Effects on the risk of cancers for example – especially those of the prostate gland, thyroid, breast and ovaries – are not yet fully understood. Some doctors therefore advise those with a family history of breast cancer or prostate cancer against taking DHEA.

DHEA raises sex hormone levels in both men and women, and the long-term effects of this are not yet clear. Some scientists also question whether taking the supplements shuts down the body's own mechanisms for producing natural DHEA. It reduces the production of luteinizing hormone (LH) in the pituitary gland for example, and prolonged use may result in lowered levels of testosterone. The long-term effects are simply unknown.

DHEA should not be taken during pregnancy, while breastfeeding or by those with acne, except under the advice of a medical practitioner. DHEA should not generally be taken under the age of 40 (unless there is a proven deficiency) as treatment may interfere with the body's natural production of the hormone.

This is obviously a controversial treatment for low sex drive. Whether or not you should take it is a decision best made with the individual advice of a doctor.

NB DHEA is classed as an anabolic androgen and is prohibited in competitive sport.

DHEA from wild yam

Some supplements labelled DHEA actually contain diosgenin, a steroid found in the Mexican wild yam. Diosgenin can be converted to DHEA in the laboratory, but this reaction cannot occur in the body itself. A study measuring DHEA and DHEA-s levels in those taking natural wild yam supplements found no change in levels of these hormones. Wild yam did, however, have a beneficial effect on blood fat levels.

Other supplements are also available that contain breakdown products obtained from diosgenin and which contain a wide range of hormone precursors. These may have a beneficial effect by increasing natural production of DHEA in the body – the research is limited. Unfortunately, the only way to find out if they can boost your own flagging sex drive is to take them for a month to see if you notice any benefit. Some may, some may not as not everyone's metabolism is efficient at converting these phytochemical precursors into DHEA.

7-keto DHEA

The body converts DHEA into sex hormones such as testosterone and oestrogen and also produces some 7-keto-DHEA, a metabolite which is more potent than DHEA. The importance of 7-keto DHEA is that it cannot be converted into sex hormones and therefore does not have an androgenic or oestrogenic action in the body. Some supplements contain just 7-keto-DHEA without the parent DHEA. This will provide many of the beneficial effects of DHEA but will not have a direct effect to increase sex drive, although it may possibly have a secondary effect as a result of promoting general feelings of wellbeing. If you are interested in the reputed longevity/immune enhancing and memory boosting benefits of DHEA, then 7-keto-DHEA is probably the best choice. If you are interested in the prosexual benefits however, 7-keto-DHEA is not the best option.

Pregnenolone

Both pregnenolone and DHEA are synthesized in the body from cholesterol. Pregnenolone is produced first, and is then converted into
DHEA as necessary. Giving supplemental pregnenolone therefore
has a similar effect to giving DHEA in that it can increase levels of
other steroids, such as testosterone, oestrogen, progesterone and
corticosteroids. If DHEA is the mother of all sex hormones, then
pregnenolone may be described as the grandmother. Pregnenolone
can also be converted directly into progesterone and is therefore
more progestogenic than DHEA.

Pregnenolone is mainly found in the adrenal glands and brain, but
is also present in other tissues such as the liver and skin. Like DHEA,
natural levels of pregnenolone peak in the late twenties to early thirties and then start to decline. By the age of 75, a person produces
60% less pregnenolone than in their thirties.

Like DHEA, pregnenolone supplements are said to have a variety
of beneficial effects, including:

- increasing a low sex drive
- promoting general feeling of wellbeing and banishing fatigue
- reducing the effects of ageing
- improving visual and auditory perception
- enhancing memory, mental acuity, alertness and awareness
- lifting a low mood
- improving the quality of sleep
- regulating immune function
- reducing the adverse effects of stress
- reducing the risks of osteoporosis and adult-onset diabetes
- helping to reduce the symptoms of arthritis, premenstrual
  syndrome, menopause and stress.

Since pregnenolone and DHEA work in harmony, some physicians prescribe small amounts of each together. Some claim that this minimises the anabolic and oestrogenic effects of DHEA, although little research is available to confirm this.

It does seem, however, that pregnenolone is less likely to have a masculinizing effect in women than DHEA as it is less likely to increase testosterone levels.

Dose

Pregnenolone is best used only under medical supervision so that blood levels can be assessed and an appropriate dose suggested. Most physicians recommend starting with a low dose of 5mg – 10mg, which may be increased to 20mg or 30mg (occasionally 50mg) if there is no obvious effect. Once benefit is obtained, a lower maintenance dose of 2mg to 5mg per day often suffices and prevents accumulation. Regular breaks in treatment – so called hormone holidays – are also recommended. New research suggests that oral hormones should be taken with food as twice as much is absorbed when digested with meals than when taken on an empty stomach.

Like DHEA, the long-term safety of taking pregnenolone hormone is not yet known. It is not usually necessary in those aged under 40 unless blood tests confirm a clinical deficiency, which may be associated with low sex drive. The possible unwanted side effects are similar to those of DHEA.

Pregnenolone should not be used during pregnancy, when breast-feeding or if oestrogen-sensitive conditions are present except under the advice of a medical practitioner.

Pregnenolone is available in a variety of formulations: pills, capsules, sublingual tablets, cream form, micronize pills, liquid and even spray.

NB pregnenolone is classed as an anabolic androgen and, although not specifically prohibited by the International Olympic Committee, should not be used by those in competitive sports as it may be prohibited under the catch-all term 'and related substances'.

Testosterone

Testosterone is the main hormone that controls libido in both men and women. If testosterone levels fall for any reason, low sex drive will therefore result. Testosterone is produced in the body from DHEA, via an intermediate chemical known as androstenedione (*see page 101* below). Testosterone production is under the control of leutinizing hormone (LH) produced in the pituitary gland. In males, 95% of testosterone hormone is produced by the testicles, with a small amount (5%) made in the adrenal glands. Healthy adult males usually produce between 4mg and 10mg testosterone per day. Highest levels occur during the teens and early twenties, and gradually reduce in later life. Testosterone secretion also varies with the time of day, and is highest in the morning and falls by 20% – 30% by the end of the day.

Small amounts of testosterone are produced in the female ovaries and adrenal glands, while some testosterone can also be produced from progesterone and DHEA hormones in both sexes. Small amounts of testosterone are converted to oestrogen in body fat stores. This effect is more pronounced in overweight males – one reason why obesity is linked with lowered sex drive in males, and why overweight boys may develop smaller genitals and less body hair at puberty.

In males, testosterone hormone is responsible for:

- maintenance of sex drive
- growth of the larynx and deepening of the voice
- growth of the penis, testes, prostate gland and scrotum

- maintenance of male patterns of hair growth, body fat distribution and muscle bulk
- production of sperm
- maintenance of erectile function
- reducing the risk of male osteoporosis
- some cardiologists now also believe testosterone reduces male risk of coronary heart disease.

Interestingly, higher testosterone levels in males seem to increase the attractiveness of their pheromones and other male odours to females.

In women, testosterone is mostly concerned with regulating libido, through interactions with DHEA, oestrogen, progesterone and by lowering levels of prolactin hormone. Testosterone levels in women aged 40 years are around half the level found in those aged 20 years. This decline in testosterone levels may account for low sex drive in some older women, as part of the so-called female androgen deficiency syndrome.

Most testosterone circulates in the blood stream bound to protein which reduces its effects. The remaining free testosterone (around 2% of the total) is the most active. Total (bound plus free) testosterone levels average 525 ng/dL in men and 30ng/dL in women. With increasing age, levels of testosterone decline in males, while relative testosterone activity increases in women as oestrogen levels fall after the menopause.

As testosterone levels fall after middle age, some men develop symptoms of tiredness, irritability, a lowering of libido and a decrease in sexual performance, excessive sweating, hot flushes and mood swings similar to that occurring at the female menopause. This has been referred to as the male menopause (andropause or viripause). Unlike the female menopause however, men do not experience a sudden drop in hormones. Their testosterone levels only fall slowly by less than 1% a year beginning around the age of 40. Research suggests that abnormally low levels of testosterone are only found in 7% of men aged 40 to 60 years, 20% of men aged 60 – 80 years and around 35% of men aged over 80 years. When symptoms – including low sex drive – occur despite normal testosterone levels, this may be due to reduced interaction between circulating testosterone and its receptors, or to more testosterone becoming bound to protein (and therefore less active) in the circulation.

Male hormone replacement therapy with testosterone is now available to treat a low sex drive associated with clinically confirmed low levels of free (unbound) testosterone which affects around one in 200 men. An estimated 4 million American males with low testosterone levels as a result of underactive testicles (hypogonadism) are currently receiving testosterone replacement therapy. Treatment aims to raise testosterone levels to normal, not to excessively high levels – and will not produce an excessive sex drive. When given to men with normal testosterone levels, it has little significant effect on sex drive. It can, however, restore libido to its previous level for those experiencing problems due to low testosterone activity.

Some doctors believe that middle-aged and older men may develop low sex drive, and lack of zest for life because, although they have normal levels of testosterone hormone, their body cells cannot interact with it as well as in their youth. They are therefore prepared to offer testosterone replacement therapy to treat low libido even where the testicles are not functioning below par. Other doctors disagree however, and place more emphasis on improving general lifestyle factors (stress, smoking, alcohol intake) instead.

Testosterone is sometimes also prescribed for post-menopausal women whose low sex drive has not responded to oestrogen replacement therapy and all other possible causes for the problem have been excluded.

Dose

Men: usually around 5mg testosterone per day. Available as tablets, capsules, skin patches applied to the skin every 24 hours, injections (two to three times a week, or once every two to three weeks), implants (replaced every six months) or gel. A sub-lingual preparation that dissolves in the mouth is under development. Beneficial effects usually occur within two weeks of starting treatment.

Women: some post-menopausal women with low sex drive may be prescribed testosterone along with oestrogen. This has been shown to increase sex drive, and provide greater satisfaction, pleasure and more intense orgasm. Possible side effects include acne, unwanted hair growth and deepening voice, however. Excessive doses may also produce flushing, sweating, vaginal itching and clitoral enlargement. The prescribing of testosterone hormone to women remains controversial. Some doctors are against it, while others feel more research is needed to understand the possible beneficial interaction of testosterone and oestrogen after the menopause.

Testosterone replacement therapy is only available on prescription, usually from specialist clinics. It should not be taken by men with a history of hormone-sensitive cancers (e.g. prostate).

Possible unwanted side effects include:

- increased aggression
- acne
- prostate enlargement
- headache
- depression
- fluid retention
- weight gain
- reduced fertility and erectile dysfunction in excess
- prolonged erection (priapism)
- abnormal production of blood cells and bleeding problems.

Testosterone should not be taken by men with prostate problems, cancer of the male breast, diabetes, high calcium levels or long-term diseases of the heart, liver or kidneys. The long-term risks of testosterone replacement therapy remain uncertain. It has been suggested that it may increase the risk of cancer of the prostate gland or liver, although this is not yet known for certain.

A synthetic androgen, mesterolone, is also available as a tablet for treating androgen deficiency and male infertility.

Dose
25mg, two to four times daily.

Testosterone levels and sex drive have also been increased by prescribing GnRH (gonadotrophin releasing hormone). This is usually secreted by the hypothalamus in the brain, and acts on the pituitary gland to release LH (luteinizing hormone) and FSH (follicle stimulating hormone) which in turn stimulates testosterone production in the male testes.

NB testosterone is classed as an anabolic androgen and is prohibited in competitive sport.

Testosterone from wild yam
Some supplements are now available that contain breakdown products obtained from the Mexican wild yam. These may have a beneficial effect by increasing natural production of testosterone in the body and are said to help increase sex drive, energy and muscle mass formation. Unfortunately, the only way to find out if they can boost your own flagging sex drive is to take them for a month to see if you notice any benefit.

Androstenedione

Androstenedione is an androgenic (masculinizing) hormone that is closely related to testosterone and DHEA. In fact, the production of testosterone and oestrogens from DHEA involves the formation of androstenedione as an intermediate step.

Androstenedione is available over the counter in the US to boost testosterone levels. It is designed for men and may be combined with extracts of Tribulus terrestris (*see page 167*).

Dose

100mg on a cyclical, three weeks on, one week off programme.

It is best not to be taken by women as it may produce masculinizing effects such as acne, excess hair growth and deepening voice. It should certainly not be taken during pregnancy or when breastfeeding. The long-term health effects of taking androstenedione (for example on the male prostate gland) remain unknown.

The supplement is popular among body-builders and athletes who take it up to an hour before a work-out. It also has a prosexual effect and may be used to boost sex drive. As an androgenic hormone, it remains controversial and is best taken under the supervision of a physician familiar with its use.

NB androstenedione is classed as an anabolic androgen and is prohibited in competitive sport.

Oestrogen

The female hormone, oestrogen, is made up of three different hormones with similar actions. These are:

● 80% oestriol – the weakest oestrogen
● 10% oestrone
● 10% oestradiol – the most powerful oestrogen.

Oestrogen is produced in the ovaries, adrenal glands, and small amounts can also be produced from circulating testosterone hormone. Women have relatively high levels of oestrogen up until the menopause, after which they fall to between one half and one third of pre-menopausal levels. Men have relatively low levels of oestrogen throughout life but the significance of these is not fully understood. Oestrogen has many different actions in females and helps to:

- control female sex drive
- regulate the menstrual cycle
- stimulate the development of eggs
- stimulate the growth and development of breast and womb tissues
- maintain tissue elasticity, especially in the skin, blood vessel walls and reproductive tract
- maintain female body shape with fat storage around the breasts, hips and thighs
- regulate mood and female behaviour patterns
- reduce the risk of hardening and furring up of the arteries, coronary heart disease, osteoporosis and possibly some forms of dementia.

During the five years before the menopause, oestrogen levels slowly start to fall until they become too low to maintain the menstrual cycle, and periods stop. The menopause is a natural phase in a woman's life when her fertility draws to a close. It usually occurs between the ages of 45 and 55 with an average of 51 years. The ovaries and adrenal glands still continue to make small levels of oestrogen after the menopause.

Some women quickly adapt to lower levels of oestrogen and notice few – if any – problems. Others find it harder to lose their oestrogen and experience unpleasant symptoms that last from one to five years – and occasionally longer.

The effects of loss of oestrogen can cause low sex drive and are also associated with a number of short-term, medium-term and long-term symptoms as follows:

Short-term Symptoms	Medium-term Symptoms	Long-term Symptoms
hot flushes	vaginal dryness	abnormal blood
night sweats	urinary symptoms	cholesterol levels
headaches	stress incontinence,	hardening and furring
tiredness	skin/hair dryness,	up of the arteries
anxiety	thinning and loss of	high blood pressure
difficulty sleeping	elasticity	increased risk of:
irritability	shrinking of breasts	stroke
mood swings	loss of female pattern	coronary heart
poor memory	of fat storage	disease
and concentration	reduced sensation in	osteoporosis
	the skin, nipples	some types of
	and genitals	dementia

Oestrogen replacement is designed to restore oestrogen levels to their pre-menopausal range and quickly relieves short-term menopausal symptoms while helping to postpone medium and long-term symptoms. It provides a synthetic oestrogen (e.g. oestradiol, mestranol, conjugated oestrogens, oestriol, oestrone, dienoestriol) and, for women who have not had a hysterectomy, a synthetic progestogen as well, to prevent the womb lining being over-stimulated.

While oestrogen HRT is not prescribed primarily to lift a flagging sex drive, it will have beneficial effects on a low libido where it is prescribed for other indications, such as:

- to prevent a premature menopause in women whose ovaries are removed
- to relieve menopausal symptoms such as hot flushes, night sweats and mood swings

- to treat vaginal dryness, discomfort or urinary leakage
- to reduce your lifetime risk of coronary heart disease
- to reduce your lifetime risk of osteoporosis.

Dose

Varies from 25 micrograms to 2mg depending on the synthetic oestrogen used and the delivery system. A variety of oestrogen formulations are available, including tablets, skin patches, skin gels, implants and vaginal creams, pessaries or ring.

The possible side effects that have been reported with HRT include:

- nausea and vomiting
- breast tenderness and enlargement
- breakthrough bleeding
- headache
- dizziness
- leg cramps or muscle pains
- increase in size of uterine fibroids
- intolerance of contact lenses
- skin reactions
- hair thinning
- increase in body or facial hair
- premenstrual syndrome
- weight gain
- increased risk of gallstones
- increased risk of abnormal blood clotting (including deep vein thrombosis and stroke)
- may increase the risk of cancers of the breast, endometrium and ovaries.

HRT is only usually prescribed for up to ten years (counting from the age of 50) however, in order to minimize any increased risk of breast cancer.

Some women are unable to take HRT. Up to one in seven women find they are unable to cope with symptoms such as fluid retention, tender breasts, nausea, headaches, skin rashes and changes similar to premenstrual syndrome. These problems usually settle down after a few cycles of treatment however. HRT should not be taken by women who:

- are pregnant or breast feeding
- have had an oestrogen-dependent cancer (e.g. of the breast) unless their doctor agrees – an increasing number of experts now feel that women who have been successfully treated for cancer and have no evidence of a recurrence can take oestrogen HRT
- have undiagnosed vaginal bleeding
- have active endometriosis
- have active blood clotting disorders
- have severe heart, liver or kidney disease.

Oestrogen HRT remains controversial and many women are unwilling or unable to take it. Other more natural ways of balancing oestrogen levels are available and may be more appropriate if low sex drive is not associated with other more severe menopausal symptoms. These include dietary and lifestyle changes and herbal extracts containing weak plant oestrogen-like substances such as black cohosh, dong quai, ginseng, pfaffia, red clover, sage and soy extracts (*see Chapter 9 on herbs and Chapter 7 on diet*).

Some doctors now believe that if a woman is taking oestrogen replacement therapy, she should also take natural progesterone (not a synthetic progestogen) as well, even if she has had a hysterectomy and is traditionally thought not to need it (see below).

Natural progesterone

Progesterone is a hormone whose main function is to maintain pregnancy. It is mainly produced from the corpus luteum (collapsed empty egg follicle after ovulation) in the second half of the menstrual cycle, although small amounts can be made by egg follicles.

In menstruating women, levels of progesterone are approximately three times higher during the first half of the menstrual cycle, than in men. During the second half of the menstrual cycle, female levels of progesterone increase dramatically by a factor of 20. During pregnancy, progesterone levels soar even higher as the hormone is also produced by the placenta.

Progesterone plays an important role in female sex drive. High levels can, in some women, increase sex drive and also have the effect of reducing the amount of oestrogen needed to encourage sexual activity. The function of natural progesterone in males is not fully understood – it may just be a precursor produced during the manufacture of testosterone from cholesterol.

After the menopause, female progesterone levels fall to as little as to 1/120 of premenopausal levels and some doctors feel strongly that it is low progesterone levels (rather than low oestrogen levels) that are linked with post-menopausal symptoms such as mood swings and osteoporosis as well as loss of sex drive. This view is controversial, however. Traditionally, progesterone has been viewed as switching off libido but this effect mainly occurs in men. Progesterone has even been prescribed to reduce testosterone levels and sexual urges in sex offenders. It may also reduce sexual attractiveness of women to men by affecting their pheromones and other odours.

Natural progesterone cannot be taken by mouth as it is quickly inactivated in the stomach and liver. Synthetic versions of progesterone – known as progestogens – have therefore been developed for oral administration. While natural progesterone may help to boost sex drive in women whose progesterone levels are low (through an unknown mechanism), synthetic progestogens usually decrease libido and also have other unwanted side effects that do not occur with natural progesterone.

Progesterone is not found in plants, but can be synthesized in the laboratory from a chemical (diosgenin) found in wild yam and from similar chemicals in soya. Wild yam itself does not contain progesterone and the human metabolism cannot make progesterone from eating wild yam extracts. Wild yam creams only contain progesterone if a synthetic, laboratory-produced progesterone is added. This is often confusingly referred to as natural progesterone as – although it is synthetically produced – it is identical to human progesterone. A less confusing terminology is nature-identical progesterone. Progesterone derived from wild yam must be used in the form of a cream (or vaginal pessaries) as it is inactive when taken by mouth.

Progesterone cream is said to support the adrenal glands, stimulate function of the liver and endocrine glands, and to balance and regulate the female reproductive system. It may be used to help low sex drive where this is linked with premenstrual syndrome and menopausal symptoms.

Dose
Cream: differs according to formulation (e.g. 10 to 30mg daily).

Progesterone is best given in cycles. If menstruating, it is usually advised for use from day 15 – day 28 of each cycle, or day 12 to 26 (different doctors prefer different regimes). For women whose periods have stopped, it is usually given for two to three weeks out of every four. When first starting to use progesterone cream, it can sensitize the body to the effects of oestrogen, leading to breast tenderness, fluid retention and vaginal bleeding in some cases. Some physicians therefore recommend reducing the dose of oestrogen (if also being taken) at first and then re-evaluating the dose after a few months. It is best to take the advice of a physician familiar with the use of natural progesterone cream.

Tests show that the amount of progesterone in over-the-counter creams can range from zero to as high as 10%. As progesterone is fat soluble, progesterone may be absorbed through the skin – it is best to apply to thin skin such as that on the inner aspects of the arms and thighs, the face, neck, upper chest and abdomen. As progesterone may accumulate in underlying fat stores, it is suggested that the cream is rubbed into a different area of the body every day. It may take two or three months of treatment before maximum beneficial effects are experienced.

Progesterone has few adverse effects. If excess is absorbed, side effects of fluid retention, bloating and weight-gain may occur.

According to one leading protagonist of natural progesterone therapy, its main side effect is a raised sex drive so that the guy across the room will get better looking – nature's way of ensuring egg and sperm meet after ovulation! Others say that progesterone therapy switches female sex drive into reverse. But while it may reduce aggressive sex drive in women, it may actually increase passive sexual receptivity.

The role of progesterone in female sex drive is a complex and controversial subject. Most women do not experience a lowered sex drive during the second half of their menstrual cycle when their progesterone levels are at their peak, and many women do not go off sex during pregnancy when progesterone levels go through the roof. The only way to know which effect progesterone replacement therapy will have on your sex drive is to try it – where indicated after the menopause – under the supervision of a physician.

Progesterone cream is available over-the-counter in the USA but is only normally available on prescription in the UK. Just as with oestrogen replacement therapy, its use remains controversial.

Tibolone

Tibolone is a synthetic, hybrid hormone that has both oestrogenic, progestogenic and weak androgenic (testosterone-like) activity. It is prescribed for menopausal symptoms once periods have stopped for at least a year. It is particularly helpful for rebooting sex drive in post-menopausal women, and many doctors are happy to prescribe it for this indication where other menopausal symptoms are also present, assuming there are no contraindications to hormone replacement therapy.

Human growth hormone

Human Growth Hormone (HGH or somatotrophin) is currently gaining interest as an anti-ageing hormone. Like DHEA, oestrogen, progesterone and testosterone, its secretion declines significantly with age so that between the ages of 20 and 60 years, daily output decreases by as much as 75%. Growth hormone replacement therapy is said to help restore hair growth and colour, reduce wrinkles, strengthen muscle and bone and regenerate organ function. It is also said to be a powerful aphrodisiac that boosts sex drive and restores sexual potency and sexuality in older males. In one trial, HGH injections given to 202 patients showed a 75% improvement in sexual potency and frequency, erections that lasted 62% longer in men and 84% improvement in energy levels. Women with menopausal symptoms also showed improvements of over 58%. Improvements were reported within one to three months and continued to improve over six months treatment.

Growth hormone is only available as injections and these are expensive. Substances that naturally help to increase secretion of HGH from the pituitary gland can produce similar beneficial effects however. These include the amino acids L-arginine (*see Chapter 6*), lysine, ornithine, glutamine and gamma-aminobutyric acid (GABA).

9

Boosting your sex drive with prosexual herbs

Phytotherapy – the use of plant extracts for healing – is one of the most rapidly advancing areas of medical research. Traditional herbs have provided orthodox medicine with many powerful drugs including aspirin (from the willow tree), digoxin (from the foxglove) and even potent new cancer treatments such as paclitaxel from the pacific yew tree. Worldwide, specialists known as ethnobotanists are continually seeking new products from amongst the traditional herbs used by native healers. The Amazon has proved to be one of the richest sources, providing a wide range of traditional remedies. Different parts of different plants are used – roots, stems, flowers, leaves, bark, sap, fruit or seeds depending on which has the highest concentration of active ingredient. In most cases, these are dried and ground to produce a powder which is made into a tea, or packed into capsules for easy swallowing.

Almost all cultural traditions in the world have favourite aphrodisiac herbs with a reputation for increasing libido and improving impotence. Different prosexual herbs work in different ways and may, for example:

- improve general physical, mental and sexual energy levels, and are therefore effective when sex drive is low due to fatigue or exhaustion

- increase sexual desire through a direct action on brain chemicals (neurotransmitters)
- increase sexual desire through a hormone-like action or by stimulating natural hormone production in the body
- raise low mood to overcome the loss of sex drive linked with depression
- increase blood flow to the reproductive organs which may produce feelings of engorgement, tingling or throbbing
- increase production of reproductive fluids, especially semen volume, which acts as a sexual trigger in the male
- stimulate erotic dreams or thoughts
- reduce sexual inhibitions
- stimulate and strengthen erection of the penis and/or clitoris
- produce a placebo effect.

Unfortunately, few clinical trials have been carried out to investigate the efficacy of herbal supplements, so not all reputed aphrodisiacs have positive evidence to support their long tradition of use. In contrast, some of these herbs are classified as drugs in some countries and may therefore be unavailable over the counter. In Canada, for example, at least 67 herbs with a prosexual function are now considered drugs, including ginkgo, gotu kola, hypericum, kava and pau d'arco.

The following herbs can all prove helpful for boosting a low sex drive. Doses vary depending on whether you are using dried preparations, tinctures or taking extracts in the form of tablets or capsules. Where possible, try to buy a product standardized to contain a known quantity of active ingredient, and always follow the dosage instructions on packets.

NB it is best to consult a qualified herbal practitioner to select the correct herbal remedy for you. Do not take any treatment without advice if you are pregnant or planning to be.

Adaptogens

An adaptogen is a substance that strengthens, normalizes and regulates all the body's systems. It has wide-ranging, beneficial actions and boosts your immunity through several different actions rather than one specific effect. This helps you adapt to a wide variety of new or stressful situations. Some adaptogens are currently being studied for use by cosmonauts in space.

Research suggests that adaptogens work by increasing the creation of energy in body cells by making the uptake of oxygen and processing of cell wastes more efficient. This encourages cell growth and increases cell survival. Supplements with adaptogen properties also contain vitamins, minerals and unique plant chemicals whose complex role in disease prevention is still being unravelled. Adaptogens have been shown to normalize blood sugar levels, hormone synthesis, the effects of stress and disrupted biorhythms.

Adaptogens seem to work best as an energy stimulant if fatigue is not directly due to excess physical exertion but to an underlying problem such as poor or irregular diet, hormone imbalance, stress or excess consumption of coffee, nicotine or alcohol. Lifestyle changes to redress the balance (e.g. stopping or cutting back on smoking) are also important to re-energize the body. When adaptogens are used together with vitamin C and the B complex, results are often improved.

Abuta (*Chondrodendron tomentosum, Cissampelos pareira; Perieria brava*)

Abuta is a beautiful, woody vine – also known as ice vine or velvet leaf – that climbs high over trees in the West Indies, Brazil and Peru. It is popular as an ornamental plant and has large leaves – often over a foot long – which may be bruised and used externally as a poultice for treating rheumatism or snake bites. The dried root and bark are taken orally and contain a variety of isoquinoline alkaloids with anti-inflammatory and possibly some anti-cancer properties.

Abuta has traditionally been used by Brazilian women to correct hormone imbalances, improve vaginal discharge, relieve period problems – especially menstrual cramps – and to treat pre-and post-natal pain. It has antispasmodic and analgesic properties that Amazonian midwives claim can prevent threatened miscarriage. It is used in Ecuador to stop excessive bleeding after childbirth, and is commonly referred to as 'the midwives' herb'. Other uses include as a general urinary and genital tonic, for treating inflammation of the testicles (orchitis), for kidney stones, cystitis, as a mild diuretic and to prevent drowsiness after meals. This may partly relate to its use as an aphrodisiac – keeping you awake and interested, when you would otherwise only want to sleep after eating a heavy meal.

Those who would benefit are women with tiredness and exhaustion, menstrual problems, vaginal discharge or whose low sex drive is associated with discomfort after childbirth.

Dose
1 – 2g solid extract, 30 — 120ml infusion. Usually only available in mixed tinctures e.g. Touchfire Hers drops for women (Life Plus) and Jaguara (Natures Remedies).

Annatto (*Bixa orellana*)
Annatto is a small tree native to Southern and Central America and the Caribbean. It becomes covered in heart-shaped pods containing an abundance of seeds, such that a mature tree can produce as many as 600 pounds of seed! Crushed seeds are soaked in water to make an orange-yellow dye that is widely used as a food colouring in margarine, cheese and other foods.

The young shoots contain a variety of essential oils, pigments, saponins and sesquiterpenes.

In Colombia and Mexico, the leaves of the annatto tree are a valued aphrodisiac that are used to make a love tea. Annatto is also used by rainforest tribes to treat diarrhoea, fever, hepatitis and skin or vaginal infections.

Dose
Little information is available.

Ashwagandha (*Withania somnifera*)
Ashwagandha is a small evergreen shrub of the nightshade family native to India, the Mediterranean and Middle east. Its Hindi name means 'sweat of a horse' as those who take it are said to attain the strength and sexual vitality of a horse. It is also known as winter cherry or Indian ginseng.

The dried root of ashwagandha contains alkaloids and a series of steroidal lactones, known as withanolides, plus alkaloids and iron.

Ashwagandha is used as a restorative tonic and adaptogen in Ayurvedic medicine, which improves resistance to stress. It reduces anxiety and promotes serenity and deep sleep, especially in those suffering from overwork or nervous exhaustion. It is also said to strengthen muscles, tendons, bones, improve concentration, boost immunity and build *ojas* – the primary energy of the body.

Its adaptogenic properties are well researched, and may be superior to ginseng in improving mental acuity, reaction time and physical performance in healthy people.

Studies suggest, for example, that ashwagandha can prevent the depletion of vitamin C and cortisol (an adrenal hormone) in subjects under stress, as well as preventing stress-related gastrointestinal ulcers. Other studies have shown that it can increase haemoglobin levels and has anti-inflammatory properties.

Ashwagandha is a renowned aphrodisiac, that improves sexual performance and is sometimes used to treat impotence. Research carried out in 1980 shows that ashwagandha can increase haemoglobin levels, reduce greying of hair and improve sexual performance –

especially during convalescence. It may be used in both men and women, but its prosexual actions are probably best for use in men.

Dose

Powdered root: 1 – 2g daily,

Capsules standardized to contain 2 – 5mg withanolides: 150 – 300 mg.

Because ashwagandha is somewhat difficult to digest, it is often taken with ginger, warm milk, honey or hot water.

No serious side effects have been reported, even with long-term use. Those who would benefit most from taking it are men whose low sex drive is associated with anaemia, long-term stress, over-work, difficulty sleeping, exhaustion, hormonal imbalances, conva-lescence or premature ageing.

Ba ji tian (*Morinda officinalis*)

Ba ji tian is a deciduous plant native to China. Its roots yield a pungent, sweet-tasting, yellow dye that contains vitamin C and a substance known as morindin.

Ba ji tian is used to strengthen yang and is a popular prosexual tonic that strengthens the erection and can help to overcome impotence, and premature ejaculation. It is also used to help treat male and female infertility and hormonal problems such as irregular menstrual cycle.

Dose

Individually prescribed.

Black cohosh (*Cimicifuga racemosa*)

Black cohosh – also known as squaw root or black snakeroot – is an herbaceous perennial with creamy-white flower spikes that is native to shady woodlands in Canada and eastern parts of the US. Insects, especially cygus bugs, avoid black cohosh which led to the plant's

Latin name (cimex = bug; fuga = to repel). The root and rhizomes are harvested in the autumn and dried for medicinal use. It has a bitter taste and when fresh, smells unpleasant. The odour disappears on drying.

Black cohosh is an adaptogen, known for its ability to help the body adapt to changing situations and is valued for its hormone and mood balancing properties. It contains a number of oestrogen-like plant hormones (phytoestrogens) including triterpene glycosides (acteine, cimicifugoside and 27-deoxyacteine) plus isoflavonoids (formononetin) and caffeic acid derivatives (isoferulic acid). Of these, formononetin is thought to be the most important.

The female menopause is associated with decreased levels of natural oestrogen which leads to increased levels of follicle-stimulating hormone (FSH) and luteinizing hormone (LH) as the brain tries to kick-start. After the menopause, FSH and LH are secreted in large and continuous quantities. Many of the symptoms of menopause are suspected to be a result of the increased levels of LH.

Black cohosh is thought to work through the hypothalamus in the brain, and lowers levels of luteinizing hormone (produced by the pituitary gland) by as much as 20%. This in turn decreases ovarian output of progesterone hormone to normalize oestrogen-progesterone balance. Black cohosh does not affect the release of prolactin hormone, or follicle stimulating hormone (FSH). It also has a direct action on centres of the brain that help to control dilation of blood vessels, so reduces menopausal symptoms of hot flushes and sweating. Interestingly, it seems to enhance blood circulation in the genitals, and some evidence suggests it causes a significant increase in weight of the uterus and ovaries as a result.

The dried root of black cohosh is mainly used as a relaxant and a uterine stimulant to treat many gynaecological symptoms associated with raised levels of progesterone such as painful or irregular periods, labour pains, sex hormone imbalances and premenstrual syndrome, in which it can reduce feelings of depression, anxiety, tension and mood swings.

As black cohosh has a normalizing effect on female sex hormones, it may be used to improve low sex drive where this is linked with hormonal imbalances, such as after childbirth, with irregular menstruation and around the time of the menopause.

Black coshosh is the most widely used and thoroughly studied natural alternative to hormone replacement therapy (HRT). Several comparison studies have shown standardized extracts of black cohosh to produce better results in relieving hot flushes, vaginal thinning and dryness, depression and anxiety compared to standard HRT (conjugated oestrogens). For 82% of patients the treatment was described as very good (41%) or good (41%). For 11% there was little therapeutic effect but the effectiveness was described as insufficient for only 7% of women taking part.

A German trial has shown that black cohosh plus hypericum (St. John's Wort) was effective in treating 78% of women with hot flushes and other menopausal problems. Most women experience significant improvement in symptoms within two to four weeks. In another study, black cohosh out-performed Valium and oestrogen HRT (Premarin) in relieving depressive moods and anxiety.

Because its unique oestrogen action does not stimulate oestrogen-sensitive tumours (and may even inhibit them) black cohosh extracts have been used in women with a history of breast cancer. The BGA, the German equivalent of the FDA in the United States, includes no contraindications or limitations of use for cimicifuga. Black cohosh therefore offers a natural alternative to treat menopausal women where HRT is contraindicated (e.g. women with a history of oestrogen-dependent cancer, unexplained uterine bleeding, liver and gallbladder disease, pancreatitis, endometriosis, uterine fibroids or fibrocystic breast disease).

Dose
Dried rhizome and roots, 0.3 – 2g daily
Black cohosh standardized to provide 27-deoxyacteine: 1-2mg twice daily.
Liquid extract: 0.3 – 2ml daily
Tincture: 2 – 4ml daily

Black cohosh should not be taken during pregnancy or when breast-feeding.

No serious side effects have been reported. Some people have experienced headaches behind the eyes, nausea, or indigestion if they have taken too much black cohosh.

Although the German Kommission E monograph recommends that treatment with cimicifuga is limited to six months, new toxicology studies suggest black cohosh may be used long-term.

Cajueiro (*Anacardium occidentale*)
Cajueiro – also known as cashew nut – is an evergreen tree related to poison ivy and the mango, which is native to tropical America. Its nut is a popular food and medicine but has a toxic lining that must first be removed.

Cajueiro nuts and fruit contain a variety of substances including terpenes, triterpenes and beta-sitosterol.

The fruit of the cajueiro (a swollen stalk from which the nut hangs like an embryo) has a sweet flavour and isconsidered an aphrodisiac in Brazil. It is widely used (together with Catuaba and Muira puama) to treat impotence. The bark is also used to make a decoction for treating vaginal discharge and is said to be contraceptive.

Dose
No information. Often made into a juice-like drink that may be drunk in large quantities.

Catuaba (*Erythroxylon catuaba; Juniperus brasiliensis; Anemopaegma mirandum*)

Catuaba – known as the tree of togetherness or the tree of love by the Tupi Indians – is one of the most successful prosexual herbs available. There are two species, one (e. catuaba) grows vigorously in the north of Brazil, and produces hardwood forests containing trees of great height and thickness with small yellow flowers and dark yellow fruits. The other grows in the centre of Brazil and develops into a large shrub. Both species are effective in boosting sex drive when a herbal tea is made from the bark and drunk three to four times per day. The tea is bitter so honey, sugar cane brandy or Stevia (a shrub whose leaves contain a substance 100 times sweeter than sugar) are usually added to improve its taste. Brazilian couples also like to drop a piece of the tree-bark into a bottle of rum and enjoy a small glass together before retiring. Dried tree bark is mainly available in the West as capsules.

The Tupi Indians first discovered the prosexual action of catuaba and sang many songs praising it. There is a famous Brazilian saying – 'Until a father reaches 60, the son is his; after that the son is catuaba's' – for the supplement is widely used to maintain potency and fertility in older males and to treat male impotence. When the Brazilian government researched 120 local remedies used as aphrodisiacs, catuaba was one of only three selected for further study, along with damiana and Muira puama.

Catuaba tree bark contains aromatic resins and non-addictive alkaloids – catuabins – that are distantly related to cocaine. It acts as a sexual stimulant and natural aphrodisiac, promoting erotic dreams and increased sexual energy in both men and women. Erotic dreams usually start within 5 – 21 days of taking extracts regularly, followed by increased sexual desire. It also improves peripheral blood flow which may be another mechanism of action in boosting sexual performance, and has been used to combat extreme exhaustion.

Interestingly, catuaba also has anti-bacterial and anti-viral properties. Research suggests it may protect against infection with the bacteria Escherichia coli and Staphylococcus aureus, and in cell cultures it has been shown to inhibit the sticking of human immunodeficiency virus (HIV) to white blood cells, the cell-killing effect of HIV and the appearance of HIV markers on infected cells.

Dose
1g on waking, and 1g on going to bed.
No evidence of unwanted side effects, even after long-term use.

Although traditionally used to enhance male sex drive, it is also effective in women. Those who would benefit most from taking catuaba are men and women with a low sex drive – especially if due to overwork or stress – and men suffering from impotence, especially in later life.

Cayenne (*Capsicum frutescens*)
Cayenne, or chilli pepper, is a perennial shrub native to Mexico, but which is now found throughout the tropics, especially Africa and India. Its scarlet fruits filled with white seed are familiar in kitchens worldwide.

Cayenne contains up to 1.5% capsaicin. The seeds also contain steroidal saponins known as capsicidins. Capsaicin is now available in a cream prescribed as a topical painkiller to relieve post-herpetic neuralgia (shooting pains that occur after shingles) and pain linked with diabetes (peripheral neuropathy).

Cayenne is widely known as a hot, spicy supplement that stimulates circulation to the hands, feet and genitals, and which promotes sweating. It is said to have aphrodisiac properties and to help maintain an erection.

It is also used to stimulate digestion, prevent infection and to treat some types of diarrhoea.

Dose

500mg – 1000mg daily; 1 – 2ml tincture.

Chaste berry (*Vitex agnus castus*)

Agnus castus – also known as the chaste tree – is a deciduous, aromatic tree with palm-shaped leaves and small lilac flowers. It is native to the Mediterranean and West Asia and was traditionally used by monks to reduce a rampant sex drive and help them remain celibate, hence its name. It may therefore seem strange that it is included in a book on how to boost sex drive. However, chaste berry is useful in boosting sex drive (and fertility) in women suffering from premenstrual syndrome or with high prolactin levels (e.g. after childbirth). It is also used in homeopathy to boost low sex drive (*see Chapter 9*).

The berries of agnus castus contain the flavonoid, casticin, and iridoid glycosides (0.3% acubin, 0.6% agnoside and 0.07% eurostoside). No constituents have been shown to have a direct hormone action in the body, however, and it is thought to work through affecting dopamine receptors in the hypothalamus/pituitary of the brain, although this is still under investigation.

One cause of low sex drive is a raised level of prolactin hormone (*see Chapter 3*), which has a powerful libido-lowering effect. Agnus castus has been shown to lower prolactin levels and may therefore improve sex drive – but probably only in women. This is because although agnus castus has been shown to significantly reduce female prolactin levels, it has a different effect in men. At low doses, agnus castus extracts increase male prolactin levels and it is not until much higher doses are taken that it starts to reduce prolactin secretion. The low doses of active ingredients obtained by men chewing fresh berries are therefore likely to reduce sex drive – hence its traditional use by monks. In higher doses however, it may have had the opposite effect by inhibiting prolactin release.

As agnus castus is thought to have an anti-androgen effect in men, by inhibiting the action of testosterone, it is not advisable for use in males, although traditionally it has been given to treat male impotence, premature ejaculation, prostatitis, and lack of sexual sensations.

German research indicates that agnus castus primarily has a progesterone-like action in women. Agnus castus has been found to decrease secretion of follicle stimulating hormone (FSH) and increase production of leutinizing hormone (LH) probably indirectly as a result of reducing prolactin secretion. Because LH stimulates ovarian secretion of progesterone, chaste tree berry indirectly boosts progesterone levels and is valuable in treating premenstrual syndrome. Studies show it is effective in relieving physical symptoms such as headaches, sore breasts, bloating and fatigue and psychological changes such as increased appetite, sweet cravings, nervousness/restlessness, anxiety, depression, mood swings and lack of concentration in 90% of cases. It takes an average of 25 days for symptoms to start improving however.

Agnus castus is also successful in increasing fertility where difficulty in conceiving is linked with low progesterone levels during the second (luteal) phase of the menstrual cycle (from ovulation to the onset of menstruation). In one study of 45 women with this form of infertility, seven became pregnant during the three month trial and 25 women had their low progesterone levels restored to normal. Treatment should be stopped as soon as pregnancy is suspected. It is also helpful for irregular periods – tending to shorten a long cycle and lengthen a short one – and for treating menopausal symptoms (especially hot flushes and night sweats) which are indirectly linked with increased levels of FSH.

Traditionally agnus castus has been used to promote breast milk flow, even though it reduces levels of the milk-stimulating hormone, prolactin. This is because, although prolactin stimulates initial production of breast milk after childbirth, levels naturally return to normal pre-pregnancy levels within 8 days after delivery. While continued suckling maintains levels at first, these still decline, so that by 3 months after delivery, milk secretion in breastfeeding mothers continues despite prolactin levels within the normal range. Early studies involving 100 nursing mothers found that those given agnus castus extracts rather than a placebo had increased milk flow and ease of milk release. Effects took several weeks to develop and this delay suggests that another action is involved, rather than any effects on prolactin hormone secretion itself. No problems were reported with the safety of agnus castus for breast fed infants.

Dose

Tablets: 500mg daily.

Extracts standardized to contain 0.5% agnuside: 175 to 225mg daily.

Liquid extract (standardized 1:1 45%): 2ml daily.

Tincture (standardized 1:3 45%) at doses of 6 to 12 mls per day.

It is usually taken as a single daily dose first thing in the morning. It is slow acting and may take a month to show effects. The average length of treatment is six months.

Vitex agnus castus is not recommended during pregnancy. It should not be taken at the same time as other hormone treatments, such as HRT and hormonal methods of contraception.

Excess can cause a crawling sensation on the skin known as formication (like ants).

Chuchuhuasi (*Maytenus krukovit; M. ebenfolia; M. macrocarpa*)

Chuchuhuasi is prepared from the root bark of a large tree. When steeped in white rum for a week, and mixed with honey, it is taken as one of the best known jungle aphrodisiacs in Columbia and Peru. Chuchuhuasi is reputed to enhance virility and to cure male impotence, whether caused by age or illness. Its most common use, however, is to relieve symptoms of rheumatism. It is also taken as a muscle relaxant, a general revitalizing tonic for both men and women, to regulate the female menstrual cycle, as an antidiarrhoeal agent and is used as an insect repellent. Some evidence suggests that Chuchuhuasi acts as an adaptogen by boosting the function of the adrenal glands, and it is traditionally given to those convalescing from bronchitis, tuberculosis and fever.

Dose
2 – 5ml tincture daily.

Damiana (*Turnera diffusa aphrodisiaca*)

Damiana is a small shrub with aromatic leaves (smelling similar to chamomile) that is native to Mexico, Texas, Central America, northern Caribbean and Namibia. It has a long tradition of use as an aphrodisiac that can be traced back to the Ancient Mayans of Central America. Its reputation is so well established that it is even reflected in the botanical name, Turnera aphrodisiaca. There is good anecdotal evidence that it deserves its reputation as a prosexual herb and when the Brazilian government researched 120 local remedies used as aphrodisiacs, damiana was one of only three selected for further study, along with catuaba and Muira puama.

The dried leaves and stems of damiana (gathered during flowering) contain arbutin, damianin, alkaloids, cyanogenic glycosides, resins, gums, betasitosterol and 1% volatile oils such as delta-cadinene and thymol.

Its volatile, aromatic oils and beta-sitosterol have a stimulatory effect on the sexual organs and a gentle, irritant effect on the urogenital tract to produce a local, stimulant effect with tingling and throbbing sensations. Its alkaloids may also boost circulation to the genital area and increase sensitivity of nerve endings in the clitoris and penis. It also increases circulation to the penis so that erections are firmer and last longer. These combined effects are said to increase sexual desire, enhance sexual pleasure and stimulate sexual performance. Some herbalists have suggested that the alkaloids in damiana could have a testosterone-like effect (similar to those in sarsaparilla) but there seems to be no research to support this. When drunk as a tea, it produces a mild euphoria and some people use it almost as a recreational drug.

Damiana also acts as a strengthening tonic for the nervous system, is a mild laxative, a urinary antiseptic, and has been used to control headache and bed-wetting. It is specifically used in cases of anxiety and depression where there is a sexual problem such as low sex drive, impotence, premature ejaculation and recurrent genital Herpes infections.

Those who would benefit most from taking it are men and women whose loss of sex drive is linked with anxiety, emotional upsets, decreased sensitivity of the genitals, difficulty achieving arousal, physical weakness, nervous exhaustion, painful periods, menstrual headaches, recurrent cystitis or constipation. Damiana is also useful for men who have erectile difficulties.

Dose
Dried herb: 1 – 4g three times a day.
Capsules: 200mg – 800mg daily.
Tincture: 2 – 5ml up to three times a day.
1 teaspoon dried leaves infused in a cup of boiling water to make a tea, three times a day.

Usually taken on an occasional basis when needed rather than regularly. Often combined with other pro-sexual herbs such as ginseng, sarsaparilla, oats or Muira puama. Damiana's power as an aphrodisiac is said to be increased when taken in a 1 to 1 mixture with saw palmetto berries.

No serious side effects have been reported from its use. Some evidence suggests that it may reduce iron absorption from the gut so should not be used long-term.

Dong quai (*Angelica sinensis; Angelica polymorpha*)

Dong quai – sometimes spelled dang gui or tang kuei – is native to China and Japan, where it is found growing in deep mountain ravines, meadows and on riverbanks. It is called Angelica as it was supposedly revealed by the Archangel Raphael as a gift with potent, magical powers. It is widely used as a tonic for women and is sometimes referred to as female ginseng. American angelica (*A. atropurpurea*) has similar medicinal properties, but European angelica (*A. archangelica*) is only used to aid digestion and circulation.

The aromatic rhizome from chinese angelica is harvested after two years growth, and may weigh up to 0.5kg. It contains oestrogen-like substances (beta-sitosterol, coumestans), coumarin (an anticoagulant) and up to 0.8% volatile oils containing more than 60 chemicals such as ligustilide, phthalide, butylidine, sesquiterpenes and carvacrol.

Chinese angelica is valued as an adaptogen with hormone and mood balancing properties. As with other plants containing weak oestrogen-like chemicals, it has a balancing effect on oestrogen levels. It competes with oestrogen receptors in the body to help damp down the effects of excess oestrogen production (e.g. some cases of premenstrual syndrome, cyclical breast pain, endometriosis, fibroids) and also provides additional oestrogen activity where natural oestrogen levels are low (e.g. at the menopause).

It may help to boost sexuality in women whose low sex drive is linked with menopausal symptoms, heavy periods, anaemia and menstrual cramps. It is said to increase blood circulation to the pelvis, supports normal ovarian function, regulates an irregular menstrual cycle and relieves period pains. It is so successful at relieving spasm of smooth muscles (such as those in the uterine wall) that one study found it was 1.7 times more effective as an analgesic than aspirin.

Dong quai is also used as a nourishing tonic for anaemia, to stimulate the circulation, and as a laxative and to improve cyclical mood swings and headaches.

Dose

Capsules standardized to 9000ppm ligustilide: 200mg three times daily.
Dried powdered root: 500mg daily.

Do not take if you have peptic ulcers, during pregnancy or when breastfeeding. No serious side effects have been reported, although it may cause a skin rash on exposure to sun in some people.

Angelica contains anticoagulant coumarins and should not be taken in large quantities. It also contains psoralene, a compound that increases skin sensitivity to sunlight. Only small quantities should be consumed.

False unicorn (*Chamaelirium luteum; Helonias dioica*)

False unicorn is perennial herb, native to North America, which is also known as blazing star and fairy wand. It was widely chewed by native American women to help prevent recurrent miscarriage.

Its root contains up to 9% of oestrogen-like steroidal saponins similar to those found in ginseng, plus glycosides such as chamaelirin and helonin.

Little research has been performed on this interesting herb, but it is said to have a prosexual function in women similar to that of ginseng. False unicorn is used to treat gynaecological problems as it has a balancing effect on oestrogen. It contains chemicals that compete with oestrogen receptors to help damp down the effects of excess oestrogen production but also provides additional oestrogen activity where natural oestrogen levels are low. It encourages a normal menstrual cycle and has been used to help prevent and treat menopausal symptoms, endometriosis, ovarian cysts, irregular or absent periods, menopausal symptoms (especially fluid retention, tiredness, backache and low mood) and osteoporosis. It is especially useful for women who have a tendency toward pelvic congestion with sensations of heaviness.

Dose
Tincture: 10 drops, three times a day.

It can take several months for false unicorn to have an effect so is usually taken for long courses. High doses can cause nausea and vomiting.

False unicorn may be beneficial for women whose low sex drive is associated with endometriosis, pelvic congestion, recurrent miscarriage or menopausal symptoms.

Fo-ti (*Polygonum multiflorum*)
Fo-ti is a perennial climber native to central and southern China. It one of the oldest Chinese tonic herbs used to prevent ageing and is known traditionally as *he shou wu*. According to ancient legend, a middle-aged impotent and childless man, Mr He, left his village and went into the mountains over 1000 years ago. He survived for several years by eating herbs, grains, fruit and the root of fo-ti. When he finally returned to his village, his friends and relatives did not recognize him. He had a youthful appearance and his hair had changed from grey to black. From then on he became known as black-haired Mr He, which in Chinese is *he shou wu*. Taking *he shou wu* also restored his virility, allowing him to father numerous children and live to the age of 130 years.

The dried roots of fo-ti are harvested when three to four years old and contain chrysophanic acid, anthraquinones (emodin, rhein) and lecithin. Raw fo-ti roots are laxative and also toxic, but curing the root – for example by boiling it for hours in black soybean broth – converts it into a highly valued tonic that has mostly lost its laxative and toxic effects.

Fo-ti is famous for its rejuvenating and revitalizing properties. It is widely used by millions of men and women in the East as a general restorative, to promote fertility, sexual function and boost a low sex drive.

Research shows it can reduce an abnormally raised cholesterol, and may have some antibiotic effects against tuberculosis and malaria. It is also used to reduce the premature greying of hair.

Dose
Tablets: 5g daily.
Tincture: 1 dropperful tincture two or three times daily.

Pills known as Shou Wu Pian are available in Chinese herbal pharmacies and the herb is sold in health food stores as Fo Ti. It is often taken together with panax ginseng.

Avoid if suffering from diarrhoea.

Those who would benefit include men and women whose low sex drive is associated with general fatigue, lack of energy, dizziness, weakness or signs of premature ageing such as greying of the hair.

Garlic (*Allium sativum*)
Garlic is a member of the lily family. Its bulbs are divided into segments known as cloves that are so popular in the kitchen that worldwide, average consumption is equivalent to one clove per individual per day. Garlic has a number of uses and is antiseptic, antibacterial, antiviral and used to treat stomach and respiratory infections. Its most important effect for post-menopausal women is its ability to reduce the risk of coronary heart disease and stroke at a time when falling oestrogen levels naturally increase their risk.

Garlic is not such an obvious aphrodisiac, but it can boost sexual stamina by increasing circulation and reducing hardening of the arteries – a common cause of impotence in men over 40. Clinical trials using standardized tablets have shown that taking garlic regularly can reduce high blood pressure, lower levels of harmful blood fats (LDL-cholesterol and triglycerides), reduce blood stickiness and improve circulation to all parts of the body, including the genitals. Regular use reduces the risk of hardening and furring up of the arteries by up to 25%, and will therefore have a long-term beneficial effect in preventing male impotence.

Used raw, it may have on off-putting effect on partners, so take in the form of enteric coated garlic powder tablets.

Dose
600 – 900mg standardized garlic powder tablets per day

Garlic products made by solvent extraction or by boiling garlic in oil are less effective than tablets made from garlic that has been freeze-dried and powdered.

Ginger (*Zingiber officinale Roscoe*)
Ginger is a perennial, tropical plant native to the jungles of Southeast Asia. It forms knobbly, thickened structures above ground known as tuberous rhizomes. These produce roots and attractive, lance-shaped green and purple leaves. Ginger has been popular in the Orient since ancient times and is one of the oldest medicinal spices known. It was taken regularly by Confucius, the great philosopher of the 5th and 4th centuries BC, who helped to make it popular in China. In Europe it rivalled pepper as the commonest imported spice during the Middle Ages.

The familiar rhizome of ginger contains pungent gingerols, shogaols (a break-down product of gingerols produced during drying), zingerone and essential oils such as lemony citral. Ginger has analgesic, antihistamine, stimulating, anti-inflammatory and anti-nauseant properties. They have a warming effect and promote sweating, which is popular for treating colds and fevers.

Ginger has long been used to ginger up a low sex drive and was mentioned in Scheherazade's *Thousand and One Nights* (dating from the 10th century AD) as an aphrodisiac. Gingerol has a similar structure to aspirin, and ginger was recently found to be at least as effective as garlic in reducing blood clotting, boosting the circulation and lowering blood pressure. It is thought to work as a prosexual supplement by increasing blood flow to the genitals, especially the penis.

Ginger is also frequently used to quell motion sickness, morning sickness during pregnancy, and to relieve migrainous headaches. It can also help to relieve indigestion, wind, diarrhoea, suppressed menstruation and poor circulation.

Dose

Fresh: Add 7.5g fresh ginger (sliced and bruised or grated) to a mug of boiling water. Steep for five minutes and add milk or honey and lemon to taste.

Powdered ginger root standardized for 0.4% volatile oils: 250mg two to four times daily.

There is no evidence of any side effects. Do not exceed recommended doses during pregnancy.

Ginkgo (*Ginkgo biloba*)

The Ginkgo biloba, or maidenhair tree, is one of the oldest known plants. It seems to have remained unchanged during the last 200 million years and is often described as a living fossil. Ginkgo trees can grow as high as 80 to 125 feet and produce characteristic fan-shaped leaves that contain powerful antioxidants, flavoglycosides, bioflavones and unique chemicals known as ginkgolides and bilob-alides. These have been found to relax blood vessels in the body and boost blood circulation to the brain, hands, feet and genitals by stop-ping cell fragments in the blood (platelets) from clumping together.

Ginkgo is a true prosexual supplement. Research shows it can improve blood flow to the penis to strengthen and maintain an erec-tion, even at a relatively low dose of 60mg daily for 12 – 18 months. Research involving males with erectile dysfunction showed a benefi-cial effect after six to eight weeks treatment, and after six months half of patients had regained full potency. In a trial involving 50 males who took ginkgo for nine months, all those who had previ-ously relied on injectable drugs to achieve an erection regained the ability to have erections. Of the 30 men who were not helped by medical drugs, 19 regained their erections with ginkgo.

Ginkgo is one of the most popular health supplements in Europe. Many people find that it helps to improve their memory and con-centration as well as easing dizziness and improving their peripheral circulation. Ginkgo biloba extracts can be used with standard anti-depressants and/or St. John's Wort for those whose low sex drive is associated with low mood – particularly in patients over 50 years of age who may also have reduced blood flow to the brain (cere-brovascular insufficiency). In one double-blind study, 40 depressed patients aged 51 to 78 years who had not benefited from standard antidepressant drugs, were given either 80mg of ginkgo biloba extract three times daily or a placebo. After eight weeks, those tak-ing ginkgo biloba showed a three fold improvement in their Hamil-ton Rating Scale for Depression (average score 14 dropped to 4.5 compared with a drop from 14 to only 13 in those taking placebo).

Ginkgo biloba extracts have also been shown to help migraine in French clinical trials, as migraine is associated with abnormal platelet clumping which ginkgo can help to correct. The daily dose in these trials ranged from 120 to 240mg.

Ginkgo is also used to treat an irregular heartbeat, varicose veins, haemorrhoids, leg ulcers, chilblains, tinnitus and anxiety.

Dose
Extracts standardized for at least 24% ginkolides: 40 – 60mg two to three times a day (take a minimum of 120mg daily). Stimulating effects last from three to six hours but effects may not be noticed until after ten days treatment.

Those who would benefit include men whose low sex drive is linked with mental fatigue, poor memory, stress during times of intensive study (e.g. for exams), peripheral vascular disease, cold extremities, chilblains, tinnitus or depression. It is also helpful for male smokers who tend to have erections that are less hard than desired (and who also need the antioxidants found in ginkgo).

It can also be used by both men and women whose low sex drive is linked with reduced sensation from the clitoris, penis or skin in general. Reduced skin sensitivity is particularly common in women after the menopause, and in one study 60% of postmenopausal women reported skin numbness compared to 20% of premenopausal women. Of these, 86.5% of women said it was a sexual problem.

Ginseng (*Panax ginseng; P. quinquefolium*)
Ginseng – usually referred to as Chinese, Korean or Asian ginseng – is a perennial plant native to North Eastern China, Eastern Russia and North Korea, which is now rare in the wild. It is a low-growing herb with pale green flowers and berries that turn red when the medicinal root is ready for harvest. High quality ginseng is collected in the autumn from plants that are five to six years old. White ginseng is produced from air-drying the root, while red ginseng (which is more potent and stimulating) is produced by steaming and then drying the root. The closely related American ginseng (P. quinque-

folius from the woodlands of east and central US and Canada) has a
similar action and is, in fact, generally preferred in Asia as it is
sweeter tasting and thought to have more yin (heat reducing capacity) than Chinese ginseng. Translated from Chinese, ginseng means
'essence of earth in the form of man'.

Ginseng contains a variety of steroidal glycosides, sterols and
saponins, known as ginsenosides, that make up 3% to 6% of the
dry root weight. Total saponin concentrations are highest in roots
from plants that are five to six years old – around the time they are
harvested. Altogether, 28 different ginsenosides have been found in
the root, stems, leaves, flowers and buds of the plant. Research suggests that American ginseng contains more of the calming and
relaxing Rb1 ginsenosides, while Korean ginseng contains more of
the stimulating Rg1 ginsenosides. Tests show that after being eaten,
ginsenosides are concentrated in the kidneys, adrenal glands, liver,
lungs, spleen, pancreas, heart, testes/ovaries and brain.

Ginseng has been used in the Orient as a revitalizing and life-
enhancing tonic for over 7000 years. It has many uses however,
which is reflected in its name – *panax* is Greek for 'cure-all'. According to legend, it was so prized that the Chinese emperors would pay
for a ginseng root with its weight in gold.

Ginseng is a true pro-sexual supplement and adaptogen, prized as
an aphrodisiac, sexual balancer and fertility enhancer. Many of the
steroidal compounds it contains are similar in structure to human
sex hormones (such as testosterone and oestrogen), and adrenocor-
ticotrophic hormone (ACTH). Ginseng seems to increase production
of ACTH from the pituitary gland in the brain, which in turn stimulates the adrenal glands to increase their output of corticosteroids
and sex hormones (usually around 5% of circulating sex hormones
such as testosterone are produced by the adrenal glands). Prelimi-
nary studies suggest that panquilon, an enzyme found in panax ginseng, is responsible for increasing sex drive.

A new explanation for the ginseng aphrodisiac effect has also been suggested. Several studies suggest it can increase levels of nitric oxide (NO) in the spongy tissue of the penis. NO is a nerve communication chemical (neurotransmitter) that is essential for a number of physiological processes, including increasing blood flow to the penis for normal erectile function and sexual arousal. This action is similar in effect to that of the new anti-impotence drug, sildenafil (Viagra). In one study, men with impotence were given either Korean red ginseng or inactive placebo for 60 days. Frequency of sexual intercourse, morning erection, firmness of penis and size of tumescence were significantly greater (67%) in those taking the ginseng than those taking placebo (28%).

Clinical trials have confirmed that ginseng helps the body adapt to physical or emotional stress and fatigue. It is stimulating and restorative, improving physical and mental energy, stamina, strength, alertness and concentration. It has a normalising effect on hormone imbalances and boosts metabolic rate. Improves peripheral circulation, including blood flow to the genitals.

Ginseng has been associated with sexual function for centuries. It has been shown to boost sexual activity and sperm production in rabbits, bulls and rats, to stimulate ovulation in hens and to prepare female rats for mating. Ginseng has been not been found to improve impotence or low sperm counts in humans, however, although it does increase desire.

Ginseng improves lung function, reduces a build up of lactic acid in exercising muscles and improves oxygen uptake in cells. Research shows that people taking ginseng have faster reaction times than those not taking it, and it improves stamina while reducing muscle cramps and fatigue. A group of hospital nurses who took ginseng were better able to stay awake and perform their night duties than those not taking it. It also lowers cholesterol levels.

Make sure you buy a good quality product from a reputable company, or one standardized to contain at least 7% ginsenosides. This will generally be more expensive, but cheap versions may contain very little active ingredient. Analysis of 50 ginseng products sold in 11 countries found that 6 contained no ginseng at all, and in the others content of ginsenosides varied from 1.9% to 9% by weight.

Dose

Depends on grade of root. Choose a standardized product, preferably with a content of at least 5% ginsenosides for American ginseng and 15% ginsenosides for Korean ginseng. Start with a low dose and work up from 200mg – 1000mg per day. Optimum dose usually around 600mg daily. It should not be taken for more than six weeks without a break. In the East, ginseng is taken in a two weeks on, two weeks off cycle. Some practitioners recommend taking it in a six weeks on, eight weeks off cycle.

Ginseng root may be grated and eaten in soups and salads, dried and powdered for use in teas and tablets, or extracts may be encapsulated in gelatin or used in vegetable oils.

Ginseng is not advised if you have high blood pressure (may make hypertension worse), glaucoma or have an oestrogen dependent condition (e.g. pregnancy, cancer of the breast, ovaries or uterus) as it contains oestrogenic compounds.

It is best to avoid taking other stimulants such as caffeine containing products and drinks while taking ginseng. Other side effects that have been reported with long-term use include sudden high blood pressure, diarrhoea, painful breasts (mastalgia), difficulty sleeping, nervousness, skin eruptions and euphoria. Together, these are known as ginseng abuse syndrome and have occurred in people taking 3g crude root every day for two years. This mimics corticosteroid poisoning and is thought to be due to over-stimulation of the adrenal or pituitary glands. High doses of 15g resulted in feelings of depersonalization and depression. Other hormonal effects, such as postmenopausal bleeding and painful breasts (mastalgia) in older women, have also been reported.

When taken in therapeutic doses in a two weeks on, two weeks off cycle, side effects should not be a problem. If you find Chinese ginseng too stimulating however, you could try American ginseng which seems to have a more gentle action.

Those who would benefit from ginseng as a prosexual supplement include men and women whose low sex drive is linked with stress, over-work, fatigue, convalescence or hormone imbalances. It is especially helpful for women experiencing menopausal symptoms.

American ginseng is said to be best for fatigue caused by nervous conditions, anxiety and insomnia, while Korean ginseng is better for fatigue with general weakness and loss of energy.

Gotu kola (*Centella asiatica or Hydrocotyle asiatica*)

Gotu kola (Centella asiatica) is an herbaceous perennial plant native to India, China, Indonesia, Australia, the South Pacific, Madagascar, and southern and middle Africa. It forms a slender, creeping plant that tends to flourish in and around water. It is reputed to increase longevity and is also referred to as the fountain of youth. Legend claims that gotu kola was used by a Chinese herbalist, Li Ching Yun, who reputedly lived to the age of 256. In Asia, many people regularly eat one leaf of gotu kola a day in the hope of prolonging their life.

The dried leaves, stems and flowers contain glycosides and triterpenoids (e.g. asiatic acid, madecassic acid, asiaticoside, and madecassoside) which are present in concentrations of 1% to 8%. Centella oil also contains glycerides of fatty acids and plant sterols such as campesterol, stigmasterol, and sitosterol. Centella samples from India, Sri Lanka, and Madagascar seem to contain different constituents however, and in India, at least three different subspecies of Centella asiatica have been found.

Gotu kola is not related to the kolanut (Cola nitida or Cola acuminata) and does not contain caffeine.

It is one of the most important Ayurvedic herbs – known as *brahmi* – prescribed to relieve anxiety and depression, improve memory, promote calm (in larger doses), relax muscle tension, boost adrenal function during times of stress and to relieve pain. It is said to have blood cleansing properties, to stop bleeding and increase physical and mental energy levels. It has also been used to treat diarrhoea, fever, absent or irregular periods, vaginal discharge and symptoms associated with varicose veins. In patients with liver cirrhosis, centella has been shown to improve the microscopic appearance of liver tissue and to reduce inflammation.

Research confirms that when used externally, it has a significant benefit in promoting healing of wounds, chronic ulcers, burns, psoriasis and keloid scars. It also improves cellulite by acting directly on fibroblasts (fibre-producing cells) to improve connective tissue structure and reduce connective tissue hardening (sclerosis).

Dose

Tincture: 0.5 – 1 dropperfuls daily.

Dried powder: 5ml two or three times daily.

Standardized extracts (usually obtained from the Madagascar variety) containing asiatic acid (30%), madecassic acid (30%), asiaticoside (40%), and madecassoside (1% to 2%): 60 to 120mg per day.

Extracts standardized to contain 25mg triterpenes: two to four capsules daily.

No serious side effects have been reported. High doses may cause headache. Large doses are calming rather than energising. Those who would most benefit are men and women needing a general energy boost and tonic or whose low sex drive is linked with anxiety, stress and excess alcohol intake.

Guarana (*Paullinia cupana*)

Guarana is a Brazilian bush that is probably the best known herbal medicine from the rain forest. The locals refer to it as the 'Food of the Gods' and use sun-dried extracts from its seeds to make a sweet, cola-like, stimulating tonic.

The dried seeds of guarana contain a complex of natural stimulants, including guaranine (a tetramethyl xanthene similar to caffeine) theobromine, theophylline, plus saponins similar to those found in Korean and American ginseng.

Guarana increases physical, mental and sexual energy levels and relieves fatigue. It is less likely to produce the irritability, poor sleep and tremor linked with excess caffeine intake as the guaranine is buffered by oily saponins that produce a natural timed-release effect. Although it acts as a stimulant, it also has a calming effect and does not usually interfere with sleep or make stress-related symptoms worse. Some people are sensitive to it however, and respond in the same way as they do to the caffeine found in coffee.

Research in Denmark has found that after taking guarana extracts for three months, volunteers had a significant increase in energy levels and reacted better to stress. It also helps to improve sexual vigour during times of stress.

In Japan, doctors advise long-distance lorry drivers to chew guarana gum to stay awake behind the wheel and as a result the number of accidents due to drivers falling asleep has significantly decreased. Guarana also seems to boost the immune system, thin the blood, reduce fluid retention, decrease appetite and raise metabolic rate. It relieves tension headache, premenstrual syndrome and period pains.

Dose

1g daily.

Guarana is available in capsules, a wine-based elixir, energy bars, Buzz Gum and as an energy drink. A single dose provides an energy boost lasting up to six hours. Choose products produced by sun-drying and grinding – roasting converts more guaranine to caffeine.

Those who would benefit most are men or women whose low sex drive is associated with physical exhaustion, tiredness or stress.

NB guarana is a restricted substance for some sports. For more information, call the Sports Council Phoneline (*See Resources*).

Horny goat weed (*Epimedium sagittatum*)

Horny goat weed – also known as lusty goatherb and *yin yang huo* – is popular in the East, but not often used in the west. It is said to make goats fornicate after eating it and is used to treat impotence and lowered fertility in men, as well as menopausal symptoms and kidney problems in women. Studies suggest that it is able to boost sperm counts and that it dilates blood vessels in the penis to increase blood flow and improve erections. It is therefore surprising that little information is available on its use.

Hypericum (*Hypericum perforatum*)

Hypericum is a perennial shrub found in many parts of the world, especially Europe and the United States. It was named Hyperikon by Hippocrates – the father of modern medicine – a name which literally means 'above an icon' as sprigs were once set above images to drive away evil spirits. It is said to have taken its common name, St. John's Wort, from the Knights of St. John of Jerusalem who used it as a salve during the Crusades. Other stories claim that its tiny red spots, symbolic of the blood of John the Baptist, appeared on the leaves of the plant on the anniversary of the saint's beheading while yet others say it is so named because its flowers always bloom on St. John's Day, June 24. 'Wort' is an old English term for plant.

Hypericum has bright yellow flowers and small oval leaves. Its other common name, thousand puncture herb, comes from the fact that when held up to the light, the petals are seen to contain numerous pinpoint red dots while the leaves reveal transparent glands resembling perforations. The glands contain a fluorescent red dye known as hypericin.

The dried leaves and flowers of St. John's Wort contain antioxidant bioflavonoids, tannins, resins, volatile oils, hypericin, pseudohypericin and hyperforin.

St. John's Wort has been used for over 2000 years to improve emotional wellbeing. It is now known to be as effective in treating mild to moderately severe depression as many prescription antidepressant drugs.

Hypericin was originally thought to inhibit a brain enzyme, (monoamine oxidase) which would increase brain levels of a number of communication chemicals (neuro-transmitters) such as serotonin and dopamine. It is now thought to work by prolonging the action of serotonin through slowing its re-uptake once it has been released. Another possibility is that it damps down the action of the chemical, interleukin–6 or IL–6. IL–6 is released by immune cells and stimulates the hypothalamus and pituitary gland in the brain to boost their output of hormones, especially those that kick-start the adrenal glands. People who are depressed usually have high levels of adrenal hormones and hypericum helps to reduce stress-induced cortisol secretion. This may partly explain its gentle effectiveness in relieving depression.

However it works, research suggests that St. John's Wort is as effective as standard antidepressant drugs for treating mild to moderately severe depression. It can lift low mood in at least 67% of those with mild to moderate depression. Studies involving over 5000 patients show that hypericum can lift mild depression within two weeks of starting the course – and the optimum effect is reached within six weeks.

Low sex drive is an early feature of depression, and hypericum can significantly boost libido where associated with depression, including seasonal affective disorder (SAD). Research in Germany involving 111 post-menopausal women (aged 45–65 years) with low sex drive plus physical exhaustion found that taking hypericum for three months helped 60% become interested in sex again, to feel sexy and to enjoy or even initiate sex with their partner. Also, 82% suffered less irritability, anxiety, low mood, hot flushes, sweating and disturbed sleep. Before the trial, 60% said they were too exhausted for sex. At the end of the trial, none felt that way. They also reported increased self-esteem, self-confidence and self respect.

Interestingly, St. John's Wort is known to inhibit pituitary secretion of prolactin (probably through its effect on IL–6). As high levels of prolactin cause a dramatic loss of sex drive, this is another way in which the herb may act as a prosexual supplement.

St. John's Wort also increases nocturnal production of melatonin hormone, to improve the quality of sleep. Studies show it reduces alpha wave and increases theta & beta brain wave frequencies and, after four weeks treatment, gives increased deep sleep phases.

Other beneficial effects include antiviral, antibacterial and anti-cancer activity which are all currently under further investigation. Certainly Herpes simplex virus types I and II as well as various strains of influenza have responded well to St. John's Wort.

Dose

Whole dried herb: 2g – 4g daily.

Extracts standardized for hypericin: 300 – 600 micrograms hypericin three times daily.

Extracts standardized to 0.3% hypericin: 300mg three times a day.

Hypericum is best taken with food.

Those who would benefit include men and women whose loss of sex drive is linked with lack of sleep, physical exhaustion, anxiety, stress, irritability, low mood, depression, recurrent Herpes simplex infection or elevated prolactin levels (e.g. after childbirth as long as you are not breastfeeding, or during treatment for prolactinoma). It is especially beneficial for those with seasonal affective disorder, recurrent brief depression and for women around the time of the menopause, and may be used together with HRT.

Side effects are significantly less likely than with standard antidepressants. Those reported include indigestion, allergic reactions, restlessness and tiredness/fatigue each in less than 1% of people.

Should not be taken during pregnancy or when breastfeeding.

Do not take together with other antidepressants, especially MAOI inhibitors, except under medical supervision.

It is best to avoid alcohol when taking hypericum.

There are no reports of skin sensitivity on exposure to sunlight (photosensitization) in therapeutic doses. Those who are sun sensitive or on medications that cause photosensitivity (e.g. tetracycline, chlorpromazine) should avoid direct skin exposure to sunlight, however – especially if fair-skinned.

Iporuru (*Alchornea floribunda*)

Iporuru is a shrub that is native to the Amazon. Its bark is harvested in the dry season when it contains a number of active ingredients including yohimbine (*see page 171*).

Yohimbine is a powerful treatment for impotence and the Tikuna Indians use iporuru to both increase fertility of females and to treat male erectile dysfunction. It seems to be taken quite widely by older men as a general tonic and aphrodisiac. Interestingly, its most popular use is to maintain joint flexibility and relieve the symptoms of osteoarthritis.

Dose

Little information available. Do not use except under medical super-vision as yohimbine can have unwanted side effects.

Kava kava (*Piper methysticum*)

Kava – sometimes referred to as kava kava – is a Polynesian peren-nial plant related to pepper. It is native to Fiji, but is widely culti-vated in Samoa, New Guinea, the Solomon Islands and elsewhere in the South Pacific. It has heart shaped leaves and a massive rootstock that can weigh as much as 10kg. Its botanical name, *Piper methys-ticum*, was given by the explorer Captain James Cook, and literally means 'intoxicating pepper'. This refers to a 3000-year-old native custom of fermenting fresh kava roots to make a potent alcoholic drink used during a variety of rituals to induce relaxation, mild euphoria, enhance dreams and to heighten sexuality. The dried root is not intoxicating however, although a few people find it produces a pleasant, dream-like state. Polynesian people refer to kava as the nourishment of the Gods and prepare it by chewing the root and then using it to make a kava tea. When chewed, the root produces an initial stinging sensation which stimulates saliva flow followed by a long-lasting numbness of the tongue and gums.

Kava root contains a variety of pyrones (e.g. kavain, methysticin, yangonin), kavalactones, flavokavins plus hormone-like sitosterol and stigmasten–4-dione–3.

Kava is widely used to combat mild anxiety as it is non-addictive and promotes feelings of relaxation and calm. It is mildly sedative, relieves muscle tension, relieves mild to moderate pain (especially due to menstrual cramps) and can also improve memory and reac-tion time. Effects are usually noticeable within a week and continue to improve over the next month. It does not alter consciousness.

A trial involving 101 patients suffering from generalized anxiety, ten-sion, agoraphobia, social phobia, insomnia and panic attacks found that kava produced an improvement in most patients within two months. By three months, the average anxiety score had dropped from 30.7 to 13.4 in those taking kava, and down to 9.9 by six months. Other studies suggest it is as effective as some prescription drugs in treating mild to moderate anxiety, and that it can significantly improve anxiety, depression and insomnia in women with menopausal symptoms.

Kava seems to work in part of the brain known as the amygdala, which regulates feelings of fear and anxiety. The amygdala is also one of the areas where benzodiazepine tranquillizers have their effect. Kava does not interact with benzodiazepine receptor sites however, and its exact action is not yet understood.

Unlike tranquillizer drugs, tests suggest that kava does not impair driving skills, co-ordination, visual perception or judgement at therapeutic doses. Exceeding recommended doses may cause problems however.

Dose
Effective doses range from 70mg and 210mg of kavalactones.
Products standardized to 70% kava lactones: 100mg three times a day.

NB some kava teas may provide over 200mg kava lactones per cup, so do not over-indulge.

Excessive use of kava at greater than recommended doses can cause dizziness, grogginess, muscle weakness and visual disturbances. High doses (400mg or more of kava lactones per day) may result in a temporary yellow discoloration of the skin or a reversible scaly skin rash known as kani. Excess can also affect liver function and is not recommended.

Do not combine kava with alcohol (may cause nausea, stomach upset or sedation), other tranquillizers, or illegal drugs. Kava should not be taken during pregnancy or when breastfeeding.

Kava should not be taken by people with Parkinson's disease as it may affect dopamine levels and produce abnormal movements.

Kava is not a true prosexual supplement, but it can improve libido in both men and women whose low sex drive is associated with anxiety, stress and difficulty relaxing or sleeping. Also useful for those with muscle tension, including back pain and stomach cramps.

Maca (*Lepidium meyenii*)

Maca is a root vegetable, related to the potato, which grows in the Peruvian Andes at heights of around 4,000m. This makes it the highest cultivated plant in the world, and it is eaten fresh, baked, or is stored and dried for later consumption when the dried roots are boiled in water or milk and mixed with honey, fruit juices and/or sugar cane rum. Maca has been used as a food staple since before the time of the Incas as it is a good source of carbohydrate, amino acids, fatty acids, vitamins B_1, B_2, B_{12}, C and E plus the minerals calcium, phosphorus, zinc, magnesium, copper and iron.

Its tubers contain a number of steroid glycosides with oestrogen-like actions, including stigmasterol, sitosterol, isothiocyanate and beta-ecdysone. Dried, powdered maca is used to increase energy and stamina and is used by some athletes as an alternative to anabolic steroids, without the side effects. It has long been reputed to act as an aphrodisiac for men and women, as an aid to female fertility and as a treatment for male impotence. It is also widely used to relieve menopausal symptoms and other gynaecological problems related to hormonal imbalances. Some researchers believe maca is superior to red Korean ginseng, and it is sometimes even referred to as Peruvian ginseng.

Dose

1g two or three times a day.

Milk thistle (Silybum marianum; Carduus marianus)

Milk thistle is a thorny, weed-like plant with purple flower-heads, that is native to Mediterranean Europe. Its leaves have distinctive white markings that according to tradition were caused by the Virgin Mary's milk.

Milk thistle seeds contain a powerful mixture of antioxidant bio-flavonoids known as silymarin, of which the most active ingredient is the flavonolignan, silibinin. Historically, milk thistle heads were boiled and eaten like globe artichoke as a spring tonic, to increase production of breast milk, as an antidepressant and to protect the liver.

More than 300 studies have shown that silymarin can protect liver cells from the poisonous effects of excess alcohol and other toxins such as those produced by death cap mushroom and chemotherapy. It works by inhibiting factors responsible for liver cell damage – free radicals and leukotrienes – and by maintaining levels of an important liver antioxidant enzyme, glutathione. Silymarin also seems to alter the outer structure of liver cell walls so poisons do not penetrate as readily. Silymarin has been shown to stimulate liver cells after viral or toxic damage by increasing the rate at which new proteins are made and by reducing fibrosis. It has also recently been shown to have a protective effect on kidney cells. As an antioxidant, silymarin is at least 200 times more potent than Vitamin C or E and is being investigated as a possible protectant against ultra-violet induced skin cancers.

Excess alcohol intake has a pronounced negative effect on sex drive by inducing enzymes that increase the breakdown of sex hormones in the liver. This lowers testosterone levels and leads to loss of sex drive, impotence, loss of vaginal secretions, menstrual problems and lowered fertility. Continued over-indulgence also leads to shrinking ovaries or testicles, reduction in penis size and loss of pubic hair. The intake that triggers these problems varies from person to person, depending on how the metabolism handles alcohol and how much exercise is taken. Weekly intakes of over 35 units for women and 50 units for men are considered dangerous and can certainly have feminising effects in males as well as increasing the risk of liver and heart damage.

Silymarin can help to improve liver function which may in turn raise testosterone levels and help to improve low sex drive where this is associated with excess alcohol.

Dose

Standardized supplements: 70mg – 200mg silymarin three times a day.

It is best to start with a low dose and slowly increase. Liver function will start to show an improvement within five days and continue over at least the next three weeks.

Those who would benefit are the estimated one in four men and one in ten women who regularly drink more than the recommended maximum intake of alcohol. Also useful for those with liver problems, those who smoke cigarettes, are exposed to environmental pollutants, use medically prescribed drugs, work in an industry where toxic chemical exposure is common, live in the country near farms where pesticides are used, do not eat an organic diet.

The only reported side effect is a mild laxative effect in some people, due to increased production of bile.

Muira puama (*Ptychopetalum olacoides; P. guyanna; Liriosma ovata*)

Muira puama – popularly known as potency wood and marapuama – is a small tree found in the Brazilian rain forest that has white flowers with an aroma similar to jasmine. Its roots, bark and wood contain resins, lupeol, campestrol and beta-sitosterol. It is widely used by natives of the Amazon and Orinoco river basins to enhance sexual desire and combat impotence.

It is widely thought to deserve its reputation as a powerful, pros-exual supplement which quickly improves libido. When the Brazilian government researched 120 local remedies used as an aphrodisiac, Muira puama was one of only three selected for further study, along with damiana and catuaba. Researchers are unsure how it works but it is thought to stimulate sexual desire both psychologically and physically, through a direct action on brain chemicals (dopamine, noradrenaline and serotonin) through stimulating nerve endings in the genitals and by boosting production/function of sex hormones, especially testosterone.

A clinical study of 262 patients found that Muira puama was more effective than yohimbine (a pharmaceutical extract from the bark of the yohimbe tree, which is an FDA-approved treatment for impotence) with 62% of subjects complaining of lack of sexual desire claiming that Muira puama had a dynamic effect on their sex lives, while 51% who had erectile dysfunction felt it was of benefit. The researchers suggested that Muira puama is one of the best herbs for treating erectile dysfunction and lack of libido.

Muira puama is also used as a general tonic for the nervous sys-tem, and is used to help treat exhaustion, neuralgia, anxiety, depres-sion, premenstrual syndrome and menstrual cramps. Interestingly, it is also said to prevent some types of baldness.

Those who would benefit include both males and females with low sex drive, and males with temporary difficulty maintaining an erection.

Dose
1 – 1.5g daily for ten to fourteen days. Most people will not need a repeat course for three to four months, unless they are over 60 when a monthly dose may be beneficial.
Tea: one cup on an occasional basis when needed
Tincture: 5ml on an occasional basis when needed.

Muira puama is often combined with other pro-sexual herbs such as ginseng, sarsaparilla and damiana. It is said to have a synergistic action with catuaba.

No serious side effects have been reported at therapeutic doses.

Nettle (*Urtica dioica*)

Stinging nettle is a perennial plant found worldwide, though few people realize it has medicinal effects. The leaves contain histamine, formic acid, acetylcholine, serotonin, glucoquinone, flavonoids, agglutinin and triterpenes while the root contains higher concentrations of beta-sitosterol and a variety of other sterols, steryl glucosides and lignans.

Nettle root extracts are taken together with saw palmetto to treat symptoms of urinary retention due to an enlarged prostate gland. The ability to improve urinary symptoms of benign prostate enlargement without shrinking the gland is a relatively new finding. Enlargement of the prostate gland in later life is linked with lower levels of the male hormone, testosterone, that occur with increasing age. The prostate gland seems to respond to falling hormone levels by enlarging to absorb more of the available hormone. Nettle extracts seem to interfere with testosterone metabolism by lowering the amount bound to a blood protein (sex hormone binding globulin – SHBG) so that more testosterone is free and active in the circulation. This means more testosterone is available for absorption into the prostate gland, so that congestion is relieved. Increased levels of freely circulating testosterone will also increase sex drive. These findings are still under investigation.

Dose

Dried extracts: 5 – 10g root extracts daily.

Tincture: 1 – 4 ml three times a day.

Dried herb: 1 – 3 teaspoons infused in boiling water three times a day.

Side effects – occasionally mild gastrointestinal upsets. Avoid over-dosage as this may cause temporary kidney problems.

NB men with prostate symptoms should continue to have a regular medical review of their condition.

Oats (*Avena sativa*)

Oat is a familiar, nutritious cereal used to make porridge and muesli. Its reputation as a prosexual herb may account for the popular saying about sowing one's wild oats.

Extracts from the young, whole plant or unripe grain, also known as oat straw or wild oats, contains saponins, flavonoids, alkaloids, steroidal compounds, vitamins (especially B group) and minerals (especially calcium).

Oatstraw is one of the most popular herbal remedies used as a restorative nerve tonic. It is recommended to help treat depression, nervous exhaustion and stress. It is a useful source of B group vitamins which are essential for energy production and which are needed in extra amounts during times of stress. Oatstraw soothes the nervous system and has a calming but spirited effect. It helps to reduce cravings and is helpful for those who are trying to stop smoking.

Research in Australia found that athletes who followed an oat-based diet for three weeks showed a 4% increase in stamina. A study involving 40 adults found that an oats and nettle supplement increased sexual desire and performance.

As oatstraw contains hormone building blocks, it is also advised for women suffering from oestrogen deficiency and for anyone with an underactive thyroid gland. Oatbran has been shown to help reduce high blood cholesterol levels and, taken regularly, can ease constipation.

Dose

1 dropperful fluid-extract or tincture two or three times daily.

People who are sensitive to gluten (coeliac disease) should allow the tincture to settle, and decant the clear liquid for use.

Those who would benefit include men and women whose low sex drive is associated with stress, exhaustion, convalescence, poor sleep, low mood or depression and who want to take a mild herb with a gentle action. Especially used at the menopause and for people with an underactive thyroid gland.

Oats may be taken during pregnancy and when breastfeeding.

Pfaffia (*Pfaffia paniculata; P. stenophylia*)

Pfaffia – also known as suma, Brazilian ginseng and Brazilian carrots – is a ground-covering vine found growing in the Brazilian mid-Atlantic forests of São Paulo and Rio de Janeiro. It is regarded as a panacea for all ills, as well as a sustaining food (roots, stems and branches) by Xingu tribesmen who call it para todo – for everything. The dried golden root of pfaffia (suma) is a rich source of vitamins, minerals, amino acids, pfaffocides and plant hormones (up to 11% by weight) such as stigmasterol and sitosterol (which have oestrogen-like actions and reduce high cholesterol levels) and beta-ecdysone which increases cellular oxygenation. It has been used as a female aphrodisiac for at least 300 years, and is also used to help treat male impotence and prostatitis.

Although pfaffia is unrelated to Chinese ginseng, it has similar adaptogenic properties and can help the immune system adapt to various stresses including overwork, illness and fatigue. It is used to boost physical, mental and sexual energy levels as well as producing a general sense of wellbeing.

Researchers have found it improves resistance to stress, illness and fatigue and evens out hormone imbalances. Due to its oestrogenic nature, it is used to treat a variety of gynaecological problems linked with hormonal imbalances such as premenstrual syndrome and menopausal symptoms – it is widely used as a natural hormone replacement therapy. The Japanese have patented an extract of the root – pfaffic acid – for its potent ability to inhibit the growth of cancer cells (melanoma). The Russians have used pfaffia at a relatively high dose as an anabolic agent to enhance muscle building without the side effects associated with banned steroids. Pfaffia is prescribed in Brazilian hospitals for cancer and diabetes, when it is taken as a tea, two or three times a day.

Pfaffocides are also being used to treat diabetes, chronic fatigue syndrome, joint problems, high cholesterol, gout and to improve sleep.

Dose

1g a day to combat physical and mental stress and as a sexual tonic. Larger doses of 15gs a day are used in treating cancer.
Extracts standardized to 5% ecdysterones: 500mg – 1gm daily.
Beneficial aphrodisiac effects are usually noticed within three to five days.

Those who would benefit include any female with a low sex drive, especially where linked with diabetes, low energy, overwork, illness, stress or chronic fatigue. Especially useful for women with premenstrual syndrome or menopausal symptoms as it has been suggested as a natural alternative to HRT. Pfaffia should not be taken during pregnancy. Although plant-oestrogens may protect against oestrogen-sensitive conditions such as endometriosis and gynaecological tumours (e.g. of the breast, ovaries and cervix) pfaffia should not be taken by women with a history of these problems except under specialist advice.

Diabetics should monitor sugar levels closely as pfaffia seems to boost insulin production, normalizes blood sugar levels and may reduce insulin requirements.

Red clover (*Trifolium pratense*)

Red clover – also known as cow clover, beebread, purple clover and trefoil – is one of over 70 different species of clover native to Europe and Asia. It has also naturalized in N. America and Australia. Of all the clovers, red clover is the most popular for medicinal use. The flower heads are collected when newly opened in spring, and the leaves and roots are also edible.

Red clover contains three classes of oestrogen-like plant hormones, isoflavones, coumestans and lignans. It is one of the few plants to contain all four isoflavones – genistein, daidzein, formononetin (methoxy-daidzein) and biochanin A (methoxy-genistein) which, plus other flavonoid glycosides, account for up to 2% dry weight.

Red clover is mainly known for its oestrogenic actions, but it also has anti-spasmodic and wound healing properties.

It is widely used to balance oestrogen levels – either where oestrogen levels are too high (by competing for stronger oestrogens in the body and diluting their effect) or by providing an additional oestrogenic boost where oestrogen levels are low. It is therefore useful for treating premenstrual syndrome, endometriosis, fibroids and meno-pausal symptoms. In one study, women past the menopause who took red clover for two weeks and followed an oestrogen-rich diet had significantly higher oestrogen levels, which then fell again when they stopped taking the supplements. Other studies have shown reduced meno-pausal symptoms of hot flushes and mood swings within three to four weeks of starting to take red clover, plus a more positive outlook on life and increased energy levels. In three clinical studies involving women with menopausal symptoms, 90% noticed such an improvement that they chose to continue treatment after the trials were completed.

Interestingly, red clover is known to have a contraceptive effect in sheep, but little information is available on its effects in human fertility.

It is also used to treat eczema, burns, psoriasis, asthma, bronchitis and some types of cancer.

Dose
500mg tablet (standardized to contain 40mg isoflavones) daily.

No serious side effects have been reported. It should not be taken during pregnancy or while breastfeeding.

Those who would benefit include women whose low sex drive is linked with oestrogen imbalances such as premenstrual syndrome, endometriosis, fibroids or menopausal symptoms.

Reishi (*Ganoderma lucidum; Ganoderma japonicum*)
Reishi is one of seven different varieties of ganoderma mushroom, each with differing colours. Reishi, which is the red ganoderma lucidum, is regarded as the superior. The Japanese refer to it as reishi (literally spiritual mushroom) while the Chinese call it *ling zhi* – the mushroom of immortality – and classify it as a superior herb equal in importance to ginseng.

Reishi has been used medicinally for over 3000 years. It is rare in the wild and until recently was only available to the nobility as it was expensive and time-consuming to gather and prepare. A recent breakthrough in organic cultivation has made it more available and therefore more affordable. The ganoderma (reishi) is grown in San Antonio under strictly sterile conditions. It is too woody and fibrous for use in the kitchen, but is widely consumed in tablet form as a herbal supplement.

Reishi contains ganodermic acids, classified as triterpenoids, which have a structure similar to steroid hormones. It also contains lentinan and a nucleotide, adenosine, which forms part of the body's energy regulation and storing system.

Reishi is a powerful adaptogen, tonic and antioxidant. It is traditionally used to strengthen the liver, lungs, heart and immune system, to increase intellectual capacity and memory, boost physical and mental energy levels and to promote vitality and longevity. It is now also used to speed convalescence, regulate blood sugar levels and to help minimize the side-effects of chemotherapy or radiotherapy. Reishi has been found to have antibacterial, anti-viral, anti-histamine, anti-allergy, anti-inflammatory (equivalent to hydrocortisone) and anti-cancer properties that are under further investigation. It also reduces blood clotting and can lower blood pressure and cholesterol levels. It has recently been shown to increase the flow of blood and oxygen uptake in the brain in people with Alzheimer's disease.

Reishi mushroom helps to bring the body's natural functions back to peak performance, including a low sex drive. It also enhances energy levels and gives a more restful night's sleep. In one Chinese study, reishi was found to relieve feelings of weariness in 78% of patients, cold extremities in 74% and insomnia in 78%. In a Japanese study of over 50 patients with essential hypertension, taking reishi extracts for six months lowered average blood pressure from 156/103 to 137/93mm Hg.

Dose
500mg two to three times daily.

Those who would benefit include those whose sex drive is linked with low energy levels, low immunity, sleep problems, chronic fatigue, stress, allergies, inflammatory problems or high blood pressure.

No serious side effects have been reported even at 300 times the therapeutic dose. A few people have experienced diarrhoea (often disappears if tablets are taken with food), irritability, thirst, dry skin rash or mouth ulcers during the first week of taking reishi.

There is no cross reaction with traditional button mushrooms and reishi can be taken by those allergic to field mushrooms.

The effects of reishi are enhanced by vitamin C which increases absorption of the active components.

Only use under medical supervision if taking immunosuppressive drugs, anticoagulants or cholesterol-lowering medication. Reishi may increase the sedative effects of certain drugs (reserpine, chlorpromazine) and inhibit the action of amphetamines.

Rye pollen (*Secale cereale*)

Extracts from the pollen of certain plants, especially rye, can reduce symptoms due to prostatitis and benign prostate enlargement. Most men (78%) with prostate problems will notice a favourable response within three months.

A double-blind, placebo-controlled study of 60 patients with BPH showed that the flower pollen extracts improved prostate symptoms by 69% compared with only 29% for those taking placebo.

The precise mode of action of flower pollen extracts is unknown. Studies suggest it damps down inflammation and inhibits 5-alpha-reductase enzyme activity to encourage shrinking of the prostate gland.

Dose

One to two 252mg tablets daily for up to eight weeks, after which you can reduce to one tablet per day for as long as required.

Rye pollen extracts are likely to be beneficial to men whose low sex drive is linked with prostate symptoms including difficulty or discomfort on passing urine, poor urinary stream and frequency, especially at night. No significant side effects have been reported.

Sage (*Salvia officinalis*)

Sage is a well-known culinary herb traditionally associated with a long, healthy life. Its leaves – especially those from the red-purple tinged varieties – contain essential oils such as borneol and camphor.

Sage is used to help reduce excessive sweating and is a popular herbal remedy for treating menopausal hot flushes and night sweats. Sage is also traditionally used to reduce the flow of breast milk during weaning, reduce excessive salivation and perspiration, soothe inflammation of the mouth, gums, throat and tongue and to soothe intestinal infections such as diarrhoea and vomiting. It can help respiratory infections such as laryngitis and tonsillitis, relieve indigestion (dyspepsia) and boost memory and concentration. It can also be applied as a compress to promote wound healing.

Dose
Sage tea: add one tablespoon of dried sage to a cup of boiling water and infuse for twenty minutes. Tincture: 2ml – 5ml.

As sage stimulates uterine contractions, it should be avoided during pregnancy, although small amounts are safe for use in cooking. It should not be used during breastfeeding unless its ability to dry up milk is required. Sage should be avoided by those with epilepsy.

Sarsaparilla (*Smilax officinalis; S. aspera; S. regelii; S. sarsaparilla; S. syphilitica* etc.)
Sarsaparilla – also popularly known as smilax – belongs to a group of climbing perennial vines that are usually armed with prickly spines. Almost four hundred different species are found in tropical and subtropical parts of the world, where the dried, thick rhizomes and slender roots are widely used medicinally. Sarsaparilla has been used as a male prosexual herb since ancient times, and was brought to Europe by Spanish traders in the 14th Century.

Sarsaparilla contains a wide range of hormone-like steroids (e.g. sarsapogenin, smilagenin, sitosterol and stigmasterol) plus their glycosides (e.g. sarsasaponin, sitosterol glucoside) that have been used commercially as the basis for synthesising sex hormones, particularly testosterone. It is therefore used by many males – especially body builders – to improve virility, vitality and energy levels. No studies have shown sarsaparilla to have an anabolic effect that increases muscle mass in humans however, and the reactions needed to convert these plant steroids into testosterone are unlikely to occur in the body. It is therefore not as virilizing as one might expect – it is even used to treat acne which is a condition usually associated with increased androgen activity.

Sarsaparilla is used to increase low sex drive in males and to help overcome impotence and infertility. Sarsaparilla is also used in lower doses in women to boost a low sex drive and improve menopausal symptoms. Because of its possible testosterone-boosting properties however, some practitioners caution against its use in women with a tendency towards excessive unwanted hair.

Sarsaparilla is mainly used as a tonic and blood purifier – it is thought to bind bacterial toxins and cholesterol in the gut so less are absorbed into the circulation. It also acts as a diuretic and promotes sweating and expectoration of catarrh. It is said to hasten regeneration and to have anti-inflammatory properties used to treat cystitis, psoriasis, eczema, acne, rheumatism, arthritis and gout, as well as infections such as syphilis, herpes, gonorrhoea and the common cold. It was surprisingly effective (90%) in curing syphilis and was included in the US Pharmacopoeia for this use from 1850 until 1950. As well as boosting hormone production in the body, sarsaparilla is said to increase the metabolic rate.

Sarsaparilla saponins seem to affect the way the body handles some prescribed drugs. In particular, it increases uptake of digitalis and increases excretion of hypnotic drugs.

It is thought to bind toxins produced by gut bacteria so these are not absorbed, reducing the work load of the liver and other organs. This may account for its use as a tonic and blood purifier.

Dose
Dried root: 1g – 4g three times a day.
Capsules: 250mg three times a day.

Liquid extract: 10ml three times a day.

No serious long-term effects have been reported. The best sarsaparilla is said to produce a slightly nauseating, acrid taste in the mouth, and even to cause a burning sensation. It may take many weeks of treatment to notice an effect on sexual function and sex drive however. Sarsaparilla can cause indigestion and, if excess is taken, may temporarily impair kidney function.

NB some dried roots labelled Mexican sarsaparilla may actually contain so-called Indian sarsaparilla, which is a different type of plant (Hemidesmus indicus) with entirely different uses. Hemidesmus is dark brown and smells of vanilla, while dried Smilax roots have a light colour (often orange tinged) and are odourless.

Saw palmetto (Sabal serrulata; Serenoa repens)

The saw palmetto is a small palm tree that is native to North America and the West Indies. It has fans of yellow-green leaves and ivory flowers that set a dark berry fruit with a nutty, vanilla flavour.

The fruit of the saw palmetto contains fatty acids, sterols (includeing ß-sitosterol, campesterol and stigmasterol), polyphrenic compounds and flavonoids.

Saw palmetto has long been hailed as a male tonic, sexual rejuvenator, aphrodisiac and is an effective treatment for shrinking an enlarged prostate gland. It is sometimes referred to as the plant catheter as it strengthens the neck of the bladder, reduces outflow obstruction due to an enlarged prostate gland, and has a diuretic action. It helps to relieve urinary discomfort, improve urinary flow and ensure better bladder voiding. In particular it controls urinary frequency and encourages shrinking of the prostate gland. Saw palmetto blocks the action of 5-alpha-reductase, a prostate enzyme that converts the male hormone, testosterone, to another hormone, dihydrotestosterone (DHT) which is linked with prostate enlargement in later life. It also inhibits another enzyme, 3-ketosteroid reductase and blocks the binding of dihydrotestosterone (DHT) to prostate cells. Saw palmetto extract has also been shown to reduce the activity of oestrogen receptors in the prostate gland. Together, these actions lower levels of DHT, help an enlarged prostate gland to shrink, and promote male sex drive by maintaining testosterone levels. It may even raise testosterone concentrations, although this effect is not yet well documented. A recent study conducted in Spain showed that the liposterolic extract of saw palmetto works by encouraging smooth muscle cell relaxation via a number of complex effects, but primarily by inhibitiing of calcium ion influx into smooth muscle cells. So, in addition to saw palmetto extract's effect on normalizing hormonal metabolism within the prostate gland, it also has a relaxant effect on the smooth muscle of the bladder neck, making it even more effective in treating benign prostatic hyperplasia (BPH).

A recent placebo-controlled study of 176 patients with BPH showed significant improvement in both day and night time urinary frequency plus a significant increase in urinary flow rate after taking saw palmetto extracts for 60 days. A randomized, controlled trial comparing extracts of saw palmetto with a prescription-only drug (finasteride) used to treat BPH showed both treatments achieved a 38% decrease in symptoms over a 6 month period. Interestingly however, sexual function in the men using the natural treatment did not change, although it deteriorated significantly in those taking the prescribed medication. Saw palmetto extracts therefore seem to be as effective as the prescribed drug for relieving symptoms of BPH, but without the undesirable side effects of low sex drive and impotence. In studies, both physicians and patients rated the efficacy of treatment as good or very good in over 80% of the cases.

Saw palmetto and nettle root are frequently combined in doses of 320mg saw palmetto and 240mg nettle root per day.

The combination of Muira puama, damiana and saw palmetto is said to work synergistically.

Saw palmetto is widely used to improve impotence and low sex drive in men. As it has oestrogenic actions, it is also used to stimulate breast enlargement in women.

Dose
Fruit extracts: 150mg – 3g daily in divided doses.
Products standardized for 85% – 95% fat-soluble sterols: 320mg daily.

Tinctures of saw palmetto do not provide significant levels of active compounds. A beneficial effect usually starts within two to six weeks. No significant side effects have been reported.

Saw palmetto is used to prevent as well as treat. It is likely to benefit men over the age of 35 by helping to prevent prostate problems, as well as older males with symptoms of prostatism (e.g. poor urinary stream, getting up at night to pass urine). Men with urinary problems should always seek medical advice for a proper diagnosis before self-treating.

Schisandra (*Schisandra chinensis*)
Schisandra – also known as magnolia vine – is an aromatic woody vine native to North-eastern China. It is a popular Chinese tonic herb also known as *wu wei zi* or five-flavoured fruit as it simultaneously tastes salty, sweet, bitter, sour and pungent. It was commonly used by Taoist women to enhance their sexual energy.

Its dried berries contain lignans such as schizandrin, phytosterols (including beta-sitosterol and stigmasterol), volatile oils and several antioxidants.

Like ginseng, schisandra has powerful adaptogenic properties and appears to be a true prosexual herb. It helps the body to adapt and cope during times of stress. It is a well-known sexual tonic that reputedly increases secretion of sexual fluids in both men and women. Schisandra berry tea is drunk in China, where the women mix it with lycii berries to increase vaginal lubrication and sexual desire. It is also taken by men to improve sexual stamina.

Schisandra has been found to increase oxygen uptake of cells and improves mental clarity, irritability, forgetfulness and prevents emotional and physical fatigue. It is regarded as a calming supplement and also boosts liver function, enhances immunity and heart function and improves allergic skin conditions such as eczema.

Dose
250mg – 500mg one to three times daily.
Dried berries: soak 5g in water overnight. Strain and brew for 15 minutes with 25ml water. Take this dose daily.

It is traditionally taken for 100 days to boost sexual energy, vitality and produce radiant skin. No serious side effects have been recorded.

Those who would benefit include both men and women whose low sex drive is linked with nervous exhaustion, general fatigue, insomnia, anxiety, excess alcohol or liver problems.

Siberian ginseng (*Eleutherococcus senticosus*)
Siberian ginseng is a deciduous, hardy shrub native to Eastern Russia, China, Korea and Japan. Its root has similar actions to that of Korean and American (panax) ginsengs, but it is not closely related. Siberian ginseng has been used in the Orient for over 2000 years. It is often regarded as an inexpensive substitute for Korean ginseng, but many researchers consider it to be a more remarkable adaptogen with a higher activity and wider range of therapeutic uses. Some users prefer it to Korean ginseng as they find it more stimulating, while others find it too strong and prefer to take the gentler American ginseng. Comparative studies suggest there is little qualitative difference

between Siberian and panax ginsengs, but eleutherococcus has the advantage of being more abundant and easier to cultivate, hence it is cheaper.

Siberian ginseng contains triterpenoid saponins known as eleutherosides, some of which are similar in structure to the saponins in panax ginseng. It is one of the most widely researched herbs, with over 1,000 scientific studies demonstrating its actions as an adaptogen that helps the body to adapt and cope during times of stress.

Siberian ginseng is widely believed to increase one's zest for life and is noted for its aphrodisiac properties. It has oestrogen-like activity and has been shown to relieve hot flushes, vaginal dryness, night sweats and anxiety. It is said to improve fertility by enhancing overall vitality and by normalising levels of sex hormones. In men, it gives higher sexual energy levels and improved ability to achieve and maintain an erection.

When given to animals, it increases milk secretion in cows, honey production by bees, and increases semen production in bulls by 28%. It also prevents wasting of the seminal vesicles (male glands that produce some seminal fluid) and prostate gland in castrated animals.

Siberian ginseng is used extensively to improve stamina and strength, particularly during or after illness and when suffering from other forms of stress and fatigue. A study involving 36 volunteers who received injections of Siberian ginseng extract three times a day for four weeks recorded a dramatic increase in numbers of immune cells, especially T-cells. Russian research suggests that as a result of boosting immunity, those taking it regularly have 40% less colds, flu and other infections compared with previous winters, and take a third fewer days off work due to health problems than those not taking it. Siberian ginseng is therefore taken by 20 million Russians every day to improve performance, wellness and adaptation to stress or change.

Siberian ginseng is also used to counter jet lag, and has been shown to help normalize high blood pressure, raised blood sugar levels and abnormal blood clotting. It is therefore used to protect against (and treat) heart disease and to promote a healthy circulation. Studies show Siberian ginseng has antibacterial properties. It is used to help recovery from radiation exposure and can improve memory and low mood. It is particularly popular with athletes as it can significantly improve performance and reaction times by decreasing lactic acid build-up in muscles, increasing glycogen storage by as much as 80%, boosting energy levels, maximising oxygen usage and speeding production of new red blood cells. In a study of 12 male athletes, those taking Siberian ginseng increased their total exercise duration by almost a quarter (23.3%), compared with only 7.5% for those taking placebo.

Dose

Siberian ginseng capsules: 1 – 2g per day. Occasionally up to 6g daily is recommended.

Tincture: 2.5 – 5ml two to three times a day for two to ten weeks.

Choose a brand that is standardized to contain more than 1% for eleutherosides.

Start with a low dose in the morning at least 20 minutes before eating. If increasing the dose, work up slowly and take two or three times per day. It is traditionally taken for two to three weeks followed by a two week break for those who are young and healthy. Those who are older, weaker or unwell may take their doses continuously.

Take on an empty stomach unless you find it too relaxing, in which case take it with meals.

Unlike Panax ginseng, Siberian ginseng does not seem to produce over-stimulation or a stress-like syndrome if excess is taken. A few people do find Siberian ginseng too strong however and it may affect their ability to sleep. If this happens, take the last dose of the day before your mid-day meal.

As with Panax ginseng, Siberian ginseng is best taken cyclically. Take daily for two to three months, then have a month without. Most people begin to notice a difference after around five days, but continue use for at least one month for the full restorative effect.

No serious side effects have been reported. Do not use (except under medical advice) if you suffer from high blood pressure, a tendency to nose bleeds, heavy periods, insomnia, rapid heart beat (tachycardia), high fever or congestive heart failure. Do not take during pregnancy or when breastfeeding except under specific medical advice.

Some practitioners maintain Siberian ginseng is good for women, while Korean (Panax) ginseng is better for men. It is really a question of trying each for a few months and deciding which suits you and your sex drive best.

Those who would benefit include men and women whose low sex drive is linked with tiredness, fatigue, depression, convalescence or exhaustion.

Tribulus terrestris

Tribulus terrestris is an Indian plant – also known as *ci ji li* – used in Ayurvedic medicine.

Its fruit contains furostanol saponins that are widely used to treat male genito-urinary problems, low sex drive and impotence. Taking tribulus for five days has been shown to increase testosterone levels in some healthy men by around 30%. A trial involving 50 male patients with low sex drive due to lethargy, fatigue and lack of interest in daily activities showed a 45% improvement in symptoms. It has diuretic actions and is traditionally used as a general male tonic, to reduce high blood pressure and as a liver stimulant.

Dose

250mg capsules standardized to contain 40% furostanol saponins.

Those who would benefit include males whose low sex drive is linked with low testosterone levels, over 45s in who testosterone levels are naturally falling, and men with erectile dysfunction.

Wild yam (Dioscorea villosa)

Wild yam is a Mexican perennial vine with heart-shaped leaves and small green flowers that is native to North and Central America. It was used medicinally by both the Maya and Aztecs to relieve colicky pain, impotence and to boost libido.

The root is rich in steroidal saponins, including dioscin, diosgenin (a break-down product of dioscin), beta-sitosterol and botogenin. Diosgenin is a hormone-like substance originally used in the laboratory to synthesize a synthetic form of progesterone (norethisterone) used in the first oral contraceptive pills. It is important to realize that wild yam does not contain progesterone, although it does seem to have progesterone-like actions. Some researchers claim that, as a herb, wild yam provides substances needed by the body to produce DHEA (*see Chapter 8*) and sex hormones such as testosterone and oestrogen. This may account for its ability to boost sex drive in both men and women. Whether or not taking wild yam can actually affect levels of human hormones is controversial however. One study involving seven volunteers (six female, one male) found no significant rises in DHEA levels even after three weeks treatment with yam. It does seem to have a progesterone-like action in the body however, and is therefore largely used as a female remedy.

Native people from the Trobriand Islands off S.E. New Guinea follow a diet that is rich in yam, other vegetables and fish. They enjoy a healthy libido and vigorous sex life yet have been noted to have fewer children than might be expected. Many researchers put this down to the natural, contraceptive action of the plant hormones found in the yam – although when taken in small quantities, it may promote female fertility where difficulty in conceiving is linked with low progesterone levels.

Wild yam acts as a general tonic and will improve mood and general feelings of wellbeing. It is also known as the colic root as it can relieve painful spasms, including painful periods, uterine contractions during labour and pain due to gallstones. It also has anti-inflammatory actions and is widely used to treat rheumatoid arthritis and diverticulitis. Research suggests that it has an antioxidant action that prevents breakdown of fatty molecules in the body (lipid peroxidation) and increases beneficial levels of HDL-cholesterol.

Dose
Capsules: 250 – 500mg powdered root:
Wild yam tea one cup daily.
Tincture: 10 – 20 drops daily.

Not to be taken in pregnancy except under medical supervision.

People who may benefit include women whose low sex drive is linked with relatively low progesterone levels such as those with pre-menstrual syndrome, menopausal symptoms or fibroids.

NB wild yam cream sold as containing natural progesterone actually contains progesterone that has been synthetically produced in the laboratory from plant-like hormones found in wild yam. It is therefore a form of hormone replacement therapy, not a herbal remedy (*see page 107*).

Yerba maté (*Ilex paraguariensis*)
Yerba maté is a tree that only grows in the rainforests of Paraguay. Sometimes just referred to as maté, its leaves, made into a tea, form a nutritional food supplement rich in vitamins and minerals – especially vitamin C. According to ancient legend, the sacred formula for preparing the leaf of yerba maté was revealed from Heaven as a

reward for faithfulness and to protect against infirmity. Missionaries have apparently gone for months at a time in the rainforests, subsisting only on yerba maté tea with no ill effects other than some weight loss. The plant must be allowed to dry for at least twelve months before use.

The leaves of yerba maté contain xanthine alkaloids – related to those in coffee and guarana – which increases mental alertness and acuity without side effects of nervousness, or sleep disturbance. It may even improve sleep patterns by normalising the amount of time spent in REM (rapid eye movement) and deep, delta-wave sleep. As a result of giving a deeper, more relaxing sleep, some users find they actually need less sleep when taking maté.

Yerba maté stimulates the adrenal glands to boost production of corticosteroids. It may therefore be classed as an adaptogen, helping the body to adapt and cope with stressful times. This effect probably also accounts for its reputed prosexual action. Many males find that drinking yerba maté tea for several days increases sexual performance.

Yerba maté is mainly used as a general energy boost, overcoming physical exhaustion and mental fatigue, especially when linked with stress. It is a popular digestive remedy which relieves indigestion and improves constipation, by both softening hard faeces and gently stimulating bowel movements, as well as a detoxifying agent that helps the elimination of wastes and toxins through both bowels and kidneys partly through a mild diuretic action.

Yerba maté is a calming tonic for anxiety, poor concentration and nervousness, lifting a low mood and relieving headaches, migraine and neuralgia. Other popular uses include strengthening heart function, lowering high blood pressure, boosting immune function and disease resistance and drying up excessive nasal secretions such as in allergic rhinitis or sinusitis. It also acts as a substitute for alcohol, and to help liver regeneration, especially when trying to reduce alcohol intake.

Those who take it claim other benefits such as increased energy levels, reduction in allergic symptoms such as hayfever, firmer and smoother skin tone and improved circulation.

Dose
Drink 2 – 3 cups Yerba maté tea per day.

Those who would benefit include men and women whose low sex drive is linked with stress, excess alcohol intake, difficulty sleeping, nervous exhaustion and general inability to cope.

As yerba maté contains high quantities of tannins, it is best not to consume it with meals as this may impair the absorption of nutrients.

Yohimbe (*Pausinystalia yohimbe; Corynanthe yohimbe*)
Yohimbe is a prosexual herbal supplement made from the bark of a tall, evergreen tree native to the West African countries of Cameroon, Gabon, Zaire and the Congo. It is one of the most potent aphrodisiac herbs, used for centuries – especially by the Bantu – to increase sexual desire, enhance sexual pleasure, boost sexual performance and treat impotence,

Yohimbe contains a mixture of up to 6% indole alkaloids, of which the main one is yohimbine. These selectively block the release of certain nerve chemicals so that small peripheral arteries dilate, increasing blood flow to the penis. These engorged arteries in turn compress the veins that carry blood away from the penis so that outflow is reduced. This results in a powerful, rigid, long-lasting erection.

Contrary to popular belief, yohimbine has no effect on testosterone levels although it does increase sex drive and physical energy levels in both men and women through an as yet ill understood action on the central nervous system, probably related to increased levels of the neurotransmitters, noradrenaline and acetylcholine.

The alkaloids in yohimbe form the basis of a drug, yohimbine hydrochloride, which is licensed for use as a treatment for male impotence in some countries. It is so successful, that 80% of men using the drug claim a good to excellent response. Because of its content of yohimbine however (and its side effects), yohimbe is classified as an unsafe herb in the US and its sale is prohibited in some states. Where it is available however, it has a powerful prosexual effect in both men and women and may promote erotic dreams.

Dose
As necessary 2.5mg. Not advised on its own, except under medical supervision.

Smaller doses of yohimbe may be contained in supplements containing other pro-sexual herbs such as ginseng, sarsaparilla, damiana and muira puama. Use only as recommended and do not exceed the stated dose.

Yohimbe is subject to legal restrictions in many countries and may, for example, be banned from sale or only available on prescription. It should only be taken on an occasional basis when needed rather than regularly. It is successful in up to one in two cases.

Unfortunately, side effects limit its use and may possibly make it dangerous for regular consumption. Adverse reactions that have been reported include anxiety, panic attacks, hallucinations, high blood pressure, increased heart rate, dizziness, headache, insomnia and skin flushing.

Yohimbe should not be used regularly. It should not be used by those with kidney disease or psychological problems – especially those taking a group of antidepressant drugs known as MAO inhibitors.

The safest way to use yohimbe is in homeopathic form, available from some specialist suppliers.

10

Boosting your sex drive with homeopathy

Homeopathy can play a helpful role in any programme to boost a low sex drive. Homeopathic medicine is based on the belief that natural substances can stimulate the body's own healing powers to relieve the symptoms and signs of illness. Natural substances are selected which, if used full-strength, would produce symptoms in a healthy person similar to those it is designed to treat. In this case, for example, substances are used that, given full strength, would lower libido. In homeopathic doses however, the opposite effect occurs and sex drive increases. This is the first principle of homeopathy, that 'like cures like'.

The second major principle of homeopathy is that increasing dilution of a solution has the opposite effect of increasing its potency, that 'less cures more'. By diluting noxious and even poisonous substances many millions of times, their healing properties are enhanced while their undesirable side effects are lost.

Homeopathic remedies are so dilute they are measured on a centesimal scale, in which dilutions of 100^{-6} are described as potencies of 6c, dilutions of 100^{-30} are written as a potency of 30c etc. To illustrate just how diluted these substances are, a dilution of 12c (100^{-12}) is comparable to a pinch of salt dissolved in the same amount of water as is found in the Atlantic Ocean!

The way in which homeopathy works is not fully understood. It is thought to have a dynamic action that boosts your body's own healing power. The principles that 'like cures like', and 'less cures more' are difficult concepts to accept, yet convincing trials have shown that homeopathy is significantly better than placebo in treating many chronic (long-term) conditions including hayfever, asthma and rheumatoid arthritis.

Homeopathic remedies should ideally be taken on their own, without eating or drinking for at least 30 minutes before or after. Tablets should also be taken without handling – tip them into the lid of the container, or onto a teaspoon to transfer them to your mouth. Then suck or chew them, don't swallow them whole.

Homeopathic treatments are prescribed according to your symptoms rather than any particular disease, so they are effective for low sex drive due to many different causes.

Homeopathic remedies may be prescribed by a medically-trained homeopathic doctor on the normal NHS prescription form and dispensed by homeopathic pharmacists for the usual prescription charge or exemptions. Alternatively, you can consult a private homeopathic practitioner or buy remedies direct from the pharmacist.

Although it is best to see a trained homeopath who can assess your constitutional type, personality, lifestyle, family background, likes and dislikes as well as your symptoms before deciding which treatment is right for you, you may find the following remedies helpful.

In most cases, you should start with a 6c potency. Treatment may be taken two or three times a day for up to a week. If partial relief occurs but the symptoms return once you stop taking the remedy, you can increase the effect by taking a 30c potency.

Some practitioners recommend that homeopathic remedies are taken for up to a week.

Sometimes, symptoms initially get worse before they get better, especially if you are using homeopathy alone. This is known as aggravation. Try to persevere as this is a good sign that the remedy is working. After completing a course of homeopathy, you will usually feel much better in yourself with a greatly improved sense of wellbeing that lets you cope with any remaining symptoms in a more positive way.

If, after taking the remedies for the time stated, there is no obvious improvement, consult a practitioner to select a remedy that is more suited to you.

NB when taking homeopathic remedies, avoid drinking strong tea or coffee if possible as these may interfere with the homeopathic effect. Similarly, you should avoid using the essentials oils of lavender, rosemary and peppermint.

Homeopathic hormones

Homeopathic hormones may be used to improve sex drive. Levels of the following hormones may be measured (e.g. in saliva) and may also be plotted over time to see how they are changing in, for example, women whose low sex drive is linked with menstrual problems or menopausal symptoms:

- oestrogen
- oestradiol
- progesterone
- testosterone
- cortisol
- DHEA
- thyroxine

Often, an imbalance is found between cortisol and DHEA levels when low sex drive is due to stress. Low sex drive is also often linked with relatively low levels of testosterone in both men and women. Homeopathic DHEA and homeopathic testosterone therefore form two important cornerstones in the homeopathic treatment of low libido by helping to regulate testosterone levels.

Homeopathic remedies for low sex drive

The following homeopathic remedies may be prescribed by a qualified practitioner depending on your symptoms and constitutional type.

Agnus castus (chaste tree)

Men: agnus castus is used where low sex drive is linked with complete lack of interest in sex and general lack of energy. It may also be used for depression, anxiety, despair and premature ejaculation – especially if sex drive was previously high.

Women: agnus castus is used where low sex drive is associated with complete lack of interest in sex – especially at the menopause, when accompanied by prolapse of the womb or when accompanied by a general lowering of energy.

Dose

6c potency, twice a day.

Amphosca

Amphosca is a complex remedy for low sex drive containing a number of homeopathic ingredients. There are two versions: one for men and one for women. They work best when both partners take a remedy (*see Resources for suppliers*).

Amphosca for Women contains: ovarinum (ovarian extract), lycopodium, selenium, damiana, agnus castus, valeriana and ambra grisea.

Amphosca for Men contains: orchitinum (testicular extract), lycopodium, selenium, damiana, agnus castus, valeriana and ambra grisea.

Arsenicum album (arsen alb: arsenic oxide)

Arsen alb is useful where low sex drive is linked with anxiety and fear of failure due to underlying insecurity and over-sensitivity. There may also be restlessness, tiredness, depression and anxiety about health.

Dose

6c potency, twice a day.

Baryta carbonica (baryta carb: barium carbonate)

Baryta carb is helpful for men with a low sex drive and so little interest in sex that they may fall asleep during intercourse. It can also be helpful for impotence when linked with low sex drive. It is especially helpful for those who lack confidence, are indecisive and who have anxiety about the size of their genitals.

Dose

6c potency, twice a day.

Bach Rescue Remedy

Bach Rescue Remedy is a homeopathic preparation designed to help men and women cope with life's ups and downs. It may be used to reduce the physical and emotional symptoms of stress and chronic illness, and to treat an emergency situation while waiting for medical assistance. Bach Rescue Remedy is especially helpful to take before intercourse for a male fearing impotence or poor performance. It can also calm the nerves of both men and women who are anticipating sex with a new partner. The remedy contains five flower essences: Cherry Plum, Clematis, Impatiens, Rock Rose and Star of Bethlehem preserved in grape alcohol (brandy). Add four drops of Rescue Remedy to a glass of water and sip slowly, every three to five minutes, holding the liquid in your mouth for a while. Alternatively, place four drops directly under your tongue.

Cactus grandiflorus (cactus grand: night-flowering cactus)

Cactus grandiflorus is useful for women whose low sex drive and aversion to sex results in painful spasm of the vaginal muscles whenever penetration is attempted (vaginismus). There may also be painful periods.

Dose

6c potency, once a day.

Calcarea carbonica (calc carb: calcium carbonate)

Calc carb is useful where low sex drive is linked with physical exhaustion, anxiety, a tendency to gain weight easily and sweat profusely. It is also useful for women with menstrual or menopausal problems.

Dose

6c potency, twice a day.

Cimicifuga (cimic: black cohosh)

Cimicifuga is useful for women whose low sex drive is linked with gynaecological problems linked with menstruation, menopause, pregnancy, postnatal depression, premenstrual syndrome or other hormone imbalances. It is especially helpful for those who are excitable, with intense emotions and strong fears.

Dose

6c potency, twice a day.

Conium maculatum (hemlock)

Conium is useful for men whose sex drive is low but still active, and linked with anxiety, erectile flaccidity or prostate enlargement. It can help those who are emotionally dulled or depressed by their lack of sexual release. Conium is also used to help those with cancer, especially of the breast. Conium is restricted for use in Australia and New Zealand.

Dose
6c potency, twice a day.

Cuprum metallicum (cuprum met: elemental copper)
Cuprum metallicum is useful for treating low sex drive that is linked with physical exhaustion and mental fatigue. It is especially helpful for those who are self-critical and with strong, unexpressed emotions which may date back to suppression of sexual urges during adolescence.

Dose
6c potency, twice a day.

Ferrum picricum (iron picrate)
Ferrum picricum is useful for men whose low sex drive is linked with prostate symptoms of urinary frequency, pain in the urethra and urinary retention.

Dose
6c potency four times a day for one month, then twice a day until symptoms improve.

Folliculinum (ovarian follicle extracts)
Folliculinum is prepared from ovarian follicle extracts and is useful for women whose low sex drive is linked with fluid retention, cyclical breast pain and mood swings.

Dose

200c potency 14 days after the start of the last period (ie day 14 of the menstrual cycle) every 12 hours for three doses. Repeat every month as necessary.

Gelsemium sempervirens (gelsemium: yellow jasmine)

Gelsemium is useful where low sex drive is associated with weariness, heavy limbs, generalized lack of energy, headaches or dizziness. It is especially helpful for those with a fear of sex that is accompanied by trembling at the thought.

Dose

6c potency, twice a day.

Graphites (graphite: pencil lead)

Men: graphites is prescribed for men whose sex drive may still be intact, but who do not indulge in intercourse because they actively dislike it. This may lead to premature ejaculation, retarded ejaculation with an uncomfortable prolongation of erection (priapism) or impotence.

Dose

6c potency, twice a day.

Women: graphites is also helpful for women with a low libido associated with dislike of sex, especially when accompanied by vaginal dryness and eczema.

Dose

6c potency, twice a day

Kali carbonicum (kali carb: potassium carbonate)

Kali carb is useful for women whose loss of sex drive is linked with exhaustion and tension after intercourse. It is especially useful for those who are possessive or who have a fear of losing control.

Dose

6c potency, twice a day.

Lachesis (bushmaster snake venom)

Lachesis is helpful where low sex drive is linked with low mood on waking which improves as the day goes on. It is also helpful for women whose low sex drive is associated with premenstrual syndrome or menopausal hot flushes.

Dose

6c potency twice a day.

Love Life

Love Life Homeopathic Tincture is a complex remedy for low sex drive containing a number of homeopathic ingredients, including agnus castus, american arum, baryta carb, cinchone, sepia, selenium, phosphorica. It is complemented by love life tablets containing a variety of oriental herbs, vitamins and minerals (see under Health of the Nation in Resources).

Lycopodium clavatum (lycopodium: club moss)

Men: lycopodium is helpful where low sex drive is linked with impotence in later life, an enlarged prostate or physical tiredness that tends to come on in the afternoon and last until the evening. It is also useful for men with an increased sex drive that is frustrated due to erectile dysfunction.

Women: lycopodium is helpful for women whose low sex drive is linked with vaginal dryness during and after intercourse. There may also be a vaginal discharge that causes burning discomfort, and/or physical tiredness that tends to come on in the afternoon and last until the evening.

Dose
6c potency, twice a day.

Moschus moschiferus (moschus: musk-deer)
Moschus is made from the sexual secretions of the musk-deer that are designed to attract females. It can be helpful where low sex drive is linked with exhaustion, fainting, anxiety about health, and over-excitability.

Dose
6c potency twice a day.

Natrum muriaticum (natrum mur: rock salt)
Natrum muriaticum is helpful for those whose low sex drive is linked with anxiety, depression and other strong emotions, especially those that are suppressed. There may also be low mood, a dislike of physical affection and a strong need to be alone. In women it is helpful where there is an aversion to sex because of vaginal discomfort and dryness.

Dose
6c potency, twice a day.

Nux vomica (nux vom: poison nut)
Nux vomica is useful for those who are workaholic and stressed, and whose low sex drive is linked with irritability, over-activity, insomnia

and excessive indulgence in alcohol, caffeine or cigarettes. It is also helpful for people who are over-sensitive, irritable and frustrated because their expectations are not being met.

Dose
6c potency, twice a day.

Phosphoricum acidum (phos. Ac: phosphoric acid)
Phos ac is one of the most effective homeopathic remedies for those whose low sex drive is linked with listlessness, lethargy, sluggishness and stress. It also takes away guilt about sex and has, for example, been used to help those distressed about masturbation, wet dreams and guilt about having sex after having a baby.

Dose
6c potency, twice a day.

Platinum metallicum (elemental platinum)
Platinum is useful for women whose low sex drive is linked with gynaecological discomfort that results in painful spasm of vaginal muscles (vaginismus) when penetration is attempted. This results in a low sex drive that stems from fear of intercourse due to pain. Women who would benefit from this remedy usually set high standards for themselves and their partners which are difficult to meet.

Dose
6c potency twice a day.

Plumbum metallicum (plumbum met: elemental lead)
Men: plumbum met is useful for men whose low sex drive is linked with hardening and furring up of the arteries, especially where this has resulted in erectile dysfunction.

Women: plumbum met is useful for women whose low sex drive and aversion to sex results in painful spasm of the vaginal muscles whenever penetration is attempted (vaginismus). There may also be breast pain and heavy periods.

Dose
6c potency, once a day.

Populace tremuloides (American aspen)
Populace tremuloides is helpful for men whose low sex drive is linked with prostate symptoms of straining to pass water and burning discomfort on urination.

Dose
6c potency four times a day for one month, then twice a day until symptoms improve.

Pulsatilla nigricans (pulsatilla: pasque flower)
Pulsatilla is useful where low sex drive is associated with weariness, physical exhaustion, weepiness and a strong need for consolation and affection. It is especially helpful for women experiencing menstrual or menopausal problems.

Dose
6c potency, twice a day.

Rhus toxicodendron (rhus tox: poison ivy)
Rhus tox is useful where low sex drive is linked with severe depression that tends to come on at night. It is especially helpful for those who are anxious, lack sensual enjoyment and who weep for no obvious reason.

Dose
6c potency, twice a day.

Sepia (sepia: cuttlefish ink)
Sepia is prescribed for a woman whose loss of sex drive and aversion to sex is severe, and linked with exhaustion, lack of motivation, indifference to sexual partners, and a tendency to become increasingly isolated, tearful and intolerant of affection. It is especially helpful for women who do not like to be touched. Symptoms may become worse premenstrually and may be linked with food cravings.

Dose
200c potency 14 days after the start of the last period (i.e. day 14 of the menstrual cycle) every 12 hours for three doses. Repeat every month as necessary.

Sepia is also used at the menopause to help relieve hot flushes and night sweats, for which the 6c or 30c potency is recommended every hour as necessary.

Staphysagria (larkspur)
Staphysagria is useful for women whose low sex drive and sexual aversion is linked with surgery (e.g. hysterectomy), unresolved anger and resentment.

Dose
6c potency, twice a day.

Sulphur (flowers of sulphur)

Men: sulphur is useful for men whose low sex drive is linked with discomfort in the penis and scrotum (especially sharp pains or itching) and erectile dysfunction.

Women: sulphur is useful for women whose low sex drive is associated with premenstrual syndrome, irritability, insomnia, lack of energy and menopausal symptoms.

Dose

6c potency, twice a day.

11

Boosting your sex drive with aromatherapy

The sense of smell has been used to stimulate sensuality for at least 4,000 years and aromatherapy was widely practised in Ancient India, Greece, Rome and Egypt. One of its most famous protagonists, Cleopatra, perfumed her body with rose, frankincense and myrrh to lure Mark Anthony. She also drenched the sails of her ship with rose oil so lovers could anticipate her floral arrival from afar. Today, modern women have professionally blended perfumes to dab behind their ears, on their wrists and in their cleavage – in fact, where ever they want to be kissed – to attract the opposite sex. Many men also use scented colognes and lotions to give their sex appeal a boost. Rather than using perfumes that contain many synthetic aromas however, you can follow the ancient practice of adorning your skin with sensual and even flagrantly erotic, natural essential oils.

Why smell is important

Every day, you breathe over 23,000 times, bringing up to 10,000 different aromatic chemicals towards receptors at the top of your nose. Their aromas are detected by hair-like nerve endings that, unlike those involved in other senses, are directly connected to your brain. Messages are passed directly to the limbic system without first being filtered by higher centres. Smells therefore have a profound effect on behaviour as they can trigger primitive responses that have not been modified by intellectual input. The limbic system is one of the most ancient parts of the brain and is linked to other nerve centres concerned with learning, memories, arousal, emotions and even hormone secretion. Smell can therefore evoke powerful responses such as hunger, nostalgia, fear and mood changes – including sexual desire. Some of these effects are triggered through the production of pheromones (*Chapter 5*).

Interestingly, the sense of smell is more acute in women than men, and is strongest around the time of ovulation. In one study of over 33 adults, women rated smell as one of the most important factors when choosing a mate. Men however considered smell and looks as being equally important when selecting a lover.

Low sex drive responds well to treatment with aromatherapy. Several different therapeutic actions may be involved, including:

- the ability to calm, relieve stress and help you relax
- mimicking the effects of natural pheromones (*see Chapter 5*)
- stimulating secretion of your own pheromones.
- stimulating erotic centres in the brain where desire originates
- releasing your inhibitions
- having an oestrogen-like effect through the plant hormones it contains
- having a testosterone-like action.

There are no essential oils that have a progesterone-like effect.

As well as stimulating the senses of others who smell the scents you are wearing – and literally increasing your animal magnetism – they also have an erotic effect on the wearer. You can therefore use aromatherapy oils to boost your own sex drive, that of your partner – or both.

When choosing an aromatherapy oil, it is essential to choose one that both you and your partner like. It is no good selecting a powerful aphrodisiac oil such as rose or jasmine if you do not like its scent for this may block its effect on your central nervous system.

What is aromatherapy?

Aromatherapy uses aromatic essential oils produced by special glands in the leaves, stems, bark, flowers, roots or seeds of many plants. These oils contain many active ingredients in a highly concentrated and potent form which, because they are volatile, readily evaporate to release their powerful scent. The oils are extracted by a variety of means. Those that are extracted by simple pressing (e.g. bergamot, lemon, orange) are known as essences, those extracted by distillation are known as essential oils, while those obtained by enfleurage (pressing petals between glass sheets coated with animal fat) and solvent extraction, are more correctly known as absolutes. Even so, the term 'essential oil' is commonly used as a catch-all phrase. Essential oils are highly concentrated and should be diluted with a carrier oil (e.g. almond, avocado, sunflower, wheatgerm oils) before use.

Aromatherapy uses a variety of techniques to obtain therapeutic benefit from these essential oils. They may be inhaled, massaged into the skin, added to bath water, or heated in a variety of ways to perfume the atmosphere and produce a therapeutic ambience. Suggestions on ways to use aromatherapy oils appear at the end of this chapter.

Oils that come into contact with skin will be absorbed to some extent and will also have a medicinal effect in the body. They can also cause irritation, and should always be diluted with a carrier oil. Excess of some oils may be harmful, so always choose oils carefully and follow the instructions that come with the pack. Never rub even diluted essential oil into the genitals as it may irritate the delicate mucus membranes and will also be super-absorbed into the body which may produce unwanted, potentially toxic effects.

Where possible, use natural rather than synthetic essential oils. Natural oils generally have a fuller, sweeter aroma that provides a greater therapeutic benefit. Also select 100% pure essential oils – these are usually more expensive but have a greater effect as they are not mixed with alcohol or other additives.

The following essential oils have properties that may help to boost your sex drive. The majority are powerful and persistent so should be used sparingly. Do not use aromatherapy essential oils during pregnancy except under the advice of a qualified aromatherapist.

Angelica

Angelica is a revitalizing yet relaxing essential oil which may be prepared from the root or seeds of the Chinese angelica, dong quai. It is one of the true prosexual essential oils and seems to have a pheromone effect that mimics that of musk. Angelica also has oestrogen–like properties and is useful for stimulating low sex drive in women with menopausal symptoms, heavy, painful or irregular periods, or who are exhausted due to anaemia. It is also beneficial to those whose low sex drive is linked with self doubt or mood swings. Angelica oil can photosensitize the skin so should not be used on any area that will be exposed to sunlight. Angelica essential oil combines well with clary-sage, cumin, geranium, rose, sandalwood and ylang-ylang.

Ambrette

Ambrette is an essential oil extracted from the seeds of the musk mallow or abelmosk (*Hibiscus abelmoschus*), which is native to India and Martinique. It is one of the true prosexual aromatherapy oils that has a warm, sensuous, musky odour. It is believed to stimulate secretion of pheromones and is an excellent prosexual oil for use by men. It combines well with black pepper, cardamom, coriander, cumin, geranium, jasmine, lemon and sandalwood.

Benzoin

Benzoin is a resin extracted from a tree, *Styrax benzoin* that is native to Thailand. It is melted down and dissolved in either ethyl glycol or wood alcohol before use. It has a woody aroma reminiscent of vanilla ice-cream and is soothing, stimulating and warming. It is one of the true prosexual aromatherapy oils that is thought to stimulate secretion of pheromones. It is useful where low sex drive is linked with self doubt, anxiety, depression, lethargy, poor circulation or premature ejaculation. Benzoin combines especially well with black pepper, cardamom, fennel, ginger, rose, rosewood, sandalwood, vanilla and ylang-ylang.

Bergamot

Bergamot essential oil is obtained from the rind of a miniature orange, *Citrus bergamia*, native to Northern Italy. The oil has a fresh, slightly spicy citrus odour that appeals to both men and women, and is familiar to many as an ingredient of Earl Grey tea. Bergamot is uplifting, relaxing and helps to release pent up emotions. It is especially helpful for those whose low sex drive is linked with mood swings, anxiety, depression or unexpressed anger. As bergamot oil photosensitizes the skin for several days, it should not be applied to any area that will later be exposed to sunlight. Bergamot blends well with cardamom, cinnamon, clary-sage, coriander, geranium, ginger, grapefruit, lavender, lemon, jasmine, juniper berry, lavender, mace, neroli, nutmeg, orange, rose, rosemary, rosewood, sandalwood, vanilla, vetiver and ylang-ylang.

Black pepper

Black pepper is a hot, spicy, sensual oil extracted from the berries of a woody, climbing plant, *Piper nigrum*, which is native to East Asia. It is a warming, stimulating oil that increases blood flow to the skin and peripheries. It is an aphrodisiac that can help to stimulate sexual desire in men or women although it is regarded as a masculine oil. Many people using it for other reasons later report a strong erotic effect, even when they were unaware of its reputation beforehand. It is useful when low sex drive is linked with fatigue, anaemia or impotence, but should not be used regularly as excess may be toxic and is irritating to the skin. A little black pepper oil added to other blends can give them a useful lift however. A green pepper oil that has a more subtle aroma may be used in the same way. Black pepper combines well with ambrette, benzoin, cumin, geranium, ginger, lemon, neroli, rosewood, sandalwood and ylang-ylang.

Cardamom

Cardamom essential oil is extracted from the seeds of a spice plant, *ellettaria cardamomum*, native to India, China and parts of the Middle East. It is related to ginger and has similar sweet, warming and aromatic properties that stimulate the appetite for food, life and sex. Many people using it for other reasons later report a strong erotic effect, even when they were unaware of its reputation as an aphrodisiac oil beforehand. It is useful when low sex drive is linked with fatigue, but should not be used regularly. Cardamom essential oil blends well with ambrette, benzoin, bergamot, coriander, fennel, jasmine, orange, rose, rosemary, rosewood, patchouli, sandalwood and ylang-ylang.

Cinnamon

Cinnamon essential oil is derived from the bark or leaves of a tree, *Cinnamomum zeylanicum*, that is native to India and Sri Lanka.

Cinnamon bark oil should not be used in any essential oil blend that will come into contact with the skin as it is classed as a hazardous oil. Cinnamon leaf oil should be used with caution for no more than a few days at a time under the supervision of a qualified aromatherapist as it may irritate the skin. Cinnamon essential oil is only included here as it may be used to perfume a room and because it has undoubted aphrodisiac actions for men. A recent study, for example, found that the smell of fresh-baked cinnamon buns consistently caused erections in the test participants. This was obviously appreciated by the ancients, who used to sprinkle cinnamon essential oil on beds before lovemaking. It combines well with a number of essential oils for use as a room perfume only. These include bergamot, coriander, ginger, jasmine, lavender, lemon, mace, neroli, nutmeg, orange, patchouli, rose, rosewood, vanilla and ylang-ylang.

Clary-sage

Clary-sage essential oil is derived from the flowers of an aromatic herb, *Salvia sclarea*, native to Italy, Syria and the South of France. It has a spicy, nutty, musky aroma that is said to resemble Muscatel wine. It is a relaxing yet uplifting oil that can produce a mild euphoria in some, but drowsiness in others. It has true aphrodisiac properties and is thought to stimulate secretion of pheromones. As it also reduces sweating, the pheromones become more concentrated on the skin. Clary-sage is also useful for helping men to overcome impotence. Although it is often thought of as a masculine oil, it appeals to many women. Clary-sage can induce colourful, erotic dreams. Do not drink alcohol if using clary-sage essential oil in aromatherapy blends however, as this can lead to nightmares. It is useful for those whose low sex drive is linked with stress, muscular tension or convalescence. Clary-sage blends well with angelica, bergamot, cumin, fennel, geranium, ginger, grapefruit, jasmine, juniper berry, lavender, lemon, neroli, nutmeg, orange, rose, rosewood, sandalwood, vetiver and ylang-ylang. Clary-sage should not be used during pregnancy.

Coriander

Coriander essential oil is derived from the seeds of a herb, *Coriandrum sativum*, native to the Far East, Spain, North Africa and Russia. The oil has a warm, fresh, spicy and slightly sweet aroma that stimulates the appetite for both food and sex. It has subtle aphrodisiac properties that are beneficial for those whose low sex drive is linked with loss of appetite, stomach cramps, low mood, mood swings, self doubt and nervous indigestion. Coriander essential oil blends well with ambrette, bergamot, cardamom, cinnamon, cumin, geranium, ginger, jasmine, lemon, mace, neroli, nutmeg, orange, rose, rosewood, vanilla and ylang-ylang.

Cumin

Cumin essential oil is derived from the seeds of a herb, *Cuminum cyminum*, that was originally native to Egypt. It has a musky, slightly bitter smell that has tonic and stimulating properties. It is one of the true prosexual aromatherapy oils and is thought to stimulate the secretion of pheromones. Cumin essential oil blends well with ambrette, angelica, black pepper, clary-sage, coriander, geranium, ginger, jasmine, neroli, rose, rosemary, rosewood, sandalwood and vanilla.

Fennel

Fennel essential oil is extracted from the seeds of a herb, *Foeniculum vulgare*, native to the Mediterranean. It is an oestrogenic herb with a warm, sensual aroma and mild diuretic properties. It is particularly useful for women whose low sex drive is linked with irregular, painful periods, premenstrual syndrome or menopausal symptoms. It can also stimulate milk flow when breastfeeding and may help to stimulate low sex drive in nursing mothers. It is useful for those under stress or in turmoil, who are finding it difficult to put their thoughts into words and who tend to over-analyze situations. Fennel essential oil blends well with benzoin, cardamom, clary-sage, geranium, lavender, lemon, nutmeg, rose, rosemary and sandalwood. Fennel should not be used for more than a few days at any one time as there is a possible risk of toxicity with excess. It should not be used during the first three months of pregnancy, or by those who suffer from epilepsy.

Geranium

Geranium essential oil is distilled from the leaves of an aromatic geranium, *Pelargonium capitatum*. It has a refreshing, exotic, slightly spicy floral scent that falls mid-way between the sweetness of rose and the sharpness of bergamot. Geranium is linked with Venus, the Roman goddess of love and is commonly used to lift a low mood and promote healing. It is said to stimulate the adrenal cortex and to balance both male and female sex hormone balance. It is a well-known aphrodisiac which has liberating, sensual properties. It is especially helpful for women whose low sex drive is linked with premenstrual syndrome, fluid retention, menopausal symptoms, mood swings, emotional turmoil or convalescence. It is also ideal for workaholics and perfectionists whose libido and emotions are damped down by their personal drive for success. Geranium combines well with most essential oils, including ambrette, angelica, bergamot, black pepper, clary-sage, coriander, cumin, fennel, juniper berry, lavender, lemon, neroli, orange, patchouli, rose, rosemary, rosewood, sandalwood, vanilla, vetiver and ylang-ylang. Geranium should not be used during pregnancy (except under the supervision of a qualified aromatherapists – some feel geranium only needs to be avoided during the first three months of pregnancy, for example). If you have sensitive skin, only use geranium oil in low concentrations.

Ginger

Ginger is an essential oil that is derived from the root/rhizome of an Asian plant, *Zingiber officinalis*. It has a hot and spicy aroma that has true aphrodisiac properties – hence the phrase to ginger up one's sex life. Women from Senegal traditionally wove belts of pounded ginger root for their husbands to wear as the aroma quickly stimulates the male sex drive. Ginger has a dynamic, fiery, sensual aroma that is beneficial for those with impotence and for men or women with total loss of sex drive. Ginger acts as a catalyst for willpower and can provide emotional support for those with loss of confidence, lack of initiative, low mood or poor determination and who tend to procrastinate. Only one or two drops are needed which is just as well as a higher concentration will irritate the skin. Ginger essential oil combines well with benzoin, bergamot, black pepper, cinnamon, clary-sage, coriander, cumin, grapefruit, jasmine, mace, nutmeg, orange, patchouli, pimento berry, rose, rosewood, sandalwood, vetiver and ylang-ylang.

Grapefruit

Grapefruit essential oil is pressed from the skin of fruits from the *Citrus paradisi* tree which is grown in many parts of the world, especially Florida, California, Brazil and Israel. It is valued for its antidepressant and diuretic properties and will form a useful part of a programme to boost sex drive in those suffering from stress, tension, irritability, low mood, especially seasonal affective disorder (SAD) and those who are over-critical of themselves and indulge in comfort eating. Grapefruit essential oil blends well with bergamot, clary-sage, ginger, juniper berry, mace, neroli, nutmeg, orange, rosewood, vanilla and ylang-ylang.

Jasmine

Jasmine is an essential oil obtained from the highly scented leaves of a climbing vine, *Jasminum officinalis*, native to India, Persia and China. It has a warm, sweet, floral aroma and is one of the true aphrodisiac essential oils. It has been revered for its powerful sensual properties for thousands of years. In India it is known as Queen of the Night – both for its heady, lingering fragrance that becomes more intense after sundown, and for its positive effects on sex drive. The Hindu god of love, Kama, tipped his arrows with jasmine blossoms to pierce the heart with desire. Jasmine is a sedative oil that has both warming and strengthening properties. It is thought to boost sex drive through a hormonal action, although some researchers believe it stimulates secretion of pheromones. Despite its inherent femininity, it is also considered to have masculine properties due to its powerful, heavy aroma. Jasmine is especially useful for impotence, women who are unable to reach orgasm and for those whose low sex drive is linked with anxiety, restlessness, low mood, lack of confidence, thoughts of inadequacy and undesirability. As a relaxant, it can help painful periods, labour pains during childbirth and, as an antidepressant is excellent for women whose low sex drive is linked with postnatal depression, especially as it can also stimulate production of breast milk. Unfortunately, it is expensive as so many jasmine petals are needed to extract just a few grams of scent. Only one or two drops are needed to add to sensual aromatherapy blends, however. Avoid cheap jasmine oils as these are either synthetic, or extracted in a way that has a lesser therapeutic effect. Jasmine essential oil combines well with ambrette, bergamot, cardamom, cinnamon, clary-sage, coriander, cumin, ginger, mace, neroli, nutmeg, orange, patchouli, pimento berry, rose, rosewood, sandalwood, vetiver and ylang-ylang. Jasmine should not be used during pregnancy (except childbirth).

Juniper Berry

Juniper Berry essential oil is extracted from the berries of a small cypress, *Juniperus communis*. Some oils are extracted from both the twigs and berries, but this has a lesser therapeutic effect, so ensure you buy one labelled juniper berry. While the oil smells strongly of turpentine, its pungent, pine wood aroma provides a pleasant smokiness in blends. Juniper Berry essential oil is a tonic, stimulating and invigorating oil that has diuretic properties. It is valuable in treating a low sex drive linked with recurrent cystitis or irregular, scanty or painful periods in women or prostate problems in men. It can help to neutralize nervous anxiety triggered by the negative emotions of others and boosts self-confidence and will power. It helps to neutralize anxiety rooted in fear of failure and is helpful for those who feel unsupported or misunderstood by others. Juniper berry combines well with bergamot, clary-sage, geranium, grapefruit, lavender, lemon, neroli, orange, rosemary and sandalwood. Juniper berry essential oil should not be used during pregnancy.

Lavender

Lavender essential oil is extracted from the flowering tops of the popular herb, *lavendula officinalis* that is native to the Mediterranean. It has a clean, refreshing smell that is calming, soothing, sedative, analgesic and antidepressant. It is useful for those whose low sex drive is linked with strong emotions, anxiety, stress, an over-active mind and insomnia. It is also helpful for those with powerful, unexpressed emotions such as fear of failure or anger and those who find it difficult to express their feelings. Lavender essential oil blends well with almost all other essences, especially bergamot, cinnamon, clary-sage, fennel, geranium, juniper berry, lemon, neroli, orange, patchouli, peppermint, pine, rosemary, rosewood, vanilla, vetiver and ylang-ylang. Lavender should be avoided during the first three months of

pregnancy. Lavender should not be used if any homeopathic remedies are being taken as it will nullify their effects.

Lemon

Lemon essential oil is expressed from the rind of the *Citrus limonum*
tree which is thought to be native to India. It has a fresh, sour, citrus
aroma that is tonic, invigorating and antidepressant. Lemon is associated with Venus, the Roman goddess of love and has long been
considered a mild aphrodisiac and is useful to sharpen the intense
sweetness of the powerful floral prosexual oils and to give them a
more masculine note for use by males. It sharpens consciousness
and clarifies the mind so is useful for those whose low sex drive is
linked with emotional fatigue, confusion, lethargy, lack of stimulation, depression and fear of emotional involvement or losing oneself
in the power of another person. Lemon essential oil blends well with
most other oils, including ambrette, bergamot, black pepper, cinnamon, clary-sage, coriander, fennel, geranium, juniper berry, lavender,
mace, neroli, nutmeg, orange, patchouli, peppermint, pine, rose,
rosemary, rosewood, sandalwood, vanilla, vetiver and ylang-ylang.
Lemon oil can photosensitize the skin so avoid subsequent exposure
to sunlight for 24 hours. Do not add more than two drops of lemon
oil to blends intended for use in the bath.

Mace

Mace essential oil is extracted from the outer, basket-like layer of the
kernel of a tree, *Myristica fragrans*, that is native to India, Java and
Sumatra. The inner kernel provides the essential oil of nutmeg.
Mace is one of the true prosexual aromatherapy oils that is thought
to stimulate the secretion of pheromones. It should only be used in
small quantities at irregular intervals. It is useful as a general aphrodisiac for both men and women. It is also useful for those whose low
sex drive is linked with lack of confidence. Mace essential oil blends

well with bergamot, cinnamon, coriander, ginger, grapefruit, jasmine,
lemon, orange, neroli, nutmeg, patchouli, pimento berry, rose, rosemary, rosewood, vanilla, vetiver and ylang-ylang.

Neroli

Neroli is a soothing essential oil extracted from the petals of the
orange tree, *Citrus aurantium*. The best quality oil comes from the
bitter Seville orange, Citrus bigaradia, which was first cultivated in
the Mediterranean. It is thought to be named after the Princess of
Neroli who first introduced the oil to Italian society in the 17th Century. Neroli has a rich, sweet, dry, floral scent that is not as citrus as
that of orange essential oil. Neroli essential oil is a calming, sedative
oil that lifts a low mood and helps to relieve feelings of tension. It is
one of the true aphrodisiac oils with a haunting bitter-sweet aroma
that calms apprehension about sex. The Romans crowned the heads
of newly-wed brides with orange blossoms to relieve wedding night
nerves. It is especially useful for those whose low sex drive is linked
with anxiety, stress and insomnia, and also in older women whose
low sex drive is linked with mood swings at the menopause. It also
helps to neutralize unexpressed emotions such as anger and resentment. Neroli essential oil blends well with bergamot, black pepper,
cinnamon, clary-sage, coriander, cumin, geranium, grapefruit,
jasmine, juniper berry, lavender, lemon, mace, neroli, orange, peppermint, rose, rosemary, rosewood, sandalwood, vanilla, vetiver and
ylang-ylang.

Nutmeg

Nutmeg essential oil is extracted from the kernel of a tree, *Myristica
fragrans*, that is native to India, Java and Sumatra. The outer basket-
like layer of the kernel provides the essential oil of mace. Nutmeg is
one of the true aphrodisiac aromatherapy oils that stimulate sensuality – possibly through a pheromone-like action. Nutmeg essential oil

combines well with bergamot, cinnamon, clary-sage, coriander, fennel, ginger, grapefruit, jasmine, lemon, mace, orange, patchouli, pimento berry, rose, rosemary, rosewood, vanilla, vetiver and ylang-ylang. Nutmeg essential oil should not be used for more than a few days at any one time as there is a possible risk of toxicity with excess. Nutmeg essential oil should not be used during pregnancy.

Orange

Orange is an essential oil extracted from the skin of the fruits of both bitter and sweet orange trees (*Citrus aurantium* species). It has similar properties to neroli, which is extracted from the orange blossoms but has an aroma that is warmer, sweeter and more citrus. It is antidepressant and mildly sedative and is useful for those whose sex drive is linked with headache, stress, frustration, depression or insomnia. It is also useful for those who work hard and strive for efficiency and perfection which may lead to frustration, irritability and tension. Only use in moderation – five or more drops added to bath water, for example, can cause skin irritation. Orange essential oil combines well with bergamot, cardamom, cinnamon, clary-sage, coriander, cumin, geranium, ginger, grapefruit, jasmine, juniper berry, lavender, lemon, mace, neroli, nutmeg, peppermint, rosemary, rosewood, vanilla, vetiver and ylang-ylang. Orange essential oil should not be used for more than a few days at any one time as there is a possible risk of toxicity with excess.

Patchouli

Patchouli is an essential oil extracted from the leaves of a bushy oriental plant, *Pogostemon patchouli*, that is native to China, Indonesia, Madagascar and Japan but widely cultivated elsewhere. It has a rich, penetrating, lingering musky, earthy odour that you either love or hate. It has a warm, calming yet stimulating scent and is one of the few aromatherapy oils to improve with age – the aroma of a patchouli oil that is more than ten years old is much more mellow and fragrant. Patchouli is one of the true prosexual aromatherapy oils that has been used as an aphrodisiac in India for thousands of years. It is thought to either mimic or stimulate secretion of pheromones. Patchouli is excellent for those who feel out of touch with their body and their sensuality, for men suffering from impotence and both men and women with a total loss of sex drive or anxiety about sex. It helps to boost libido by reducing anxiety and stress which often lead to sexual disinterest – but it will only work if used at normal strength if both partners like its strong smell. Just one drop added to blends of other essential oils can give a mysterious yet subtle oriental note without being unpleasant – even for those who dislike it. It is relaxing, energising and also anti-depressant and is said to awaken the urge to conceive. Patchouli oil blends well with bergamot, cardamom, cinnamon, geranium, ginger, jasmine, lavender, lemon, mace, nutmeg, rose, rosemary, rosewood, sandalwood and ylang-ylang.

Peppermint

Peppermint is an essential oil derived from the leaves of a common garden herb, *Mentha piperata*. It is a warming, stimulating oil best known to stimulate digestion and to help the common cold. Peppermint has an uplifting, energising and clearing effect on the mind, helping you to feel fresh and bright. This can help to boost a low sex drive linked with muddled thoughts, physical and emotional tiredness, and general feelings of lassitude and headache. As it helps to increase tolerance and receptive qualities, it is useful for helping partners to understand and accept their loved one's low sex drive. Peppermint essential oil blends well with lavender, lemon, orange, neroli, rosemary and rosewood. Only one or two drops of peppermint oil should be included in any blend as it will otherwise prove overpowering. Do not use more than three or four drops in a carrier oil blend added to a bath as this may produce a tingling sensation on the skin. Peppermint should not be used if any homeopathic remedies are being taken as it will nullify their effects. It is also best avoided in the evenings as it may interfere with sleep. Peppermint essential oil should not be used during pregnancy.

Pimento berry

Pimento essential oil is extracted from the berries of a tree, *Pimena dioica*, which is native to the West Indies and South America. It is also known as Allspice as its warm, comforting aroma resembles that of several spices – cinnamon, clove, nutmeg – mixed together. Avoid pimento oil extracted from the leaves as it is more likely to irritate the skin. The oil from the berries is one of the true prosexual aromatherapy oils that seems to stimulate secretion of pheromones. Only a single drop is needed in blends for a powerful effect – it combines particularly well with ginger, jasmine, mace and nutmeg.

Pine

Pine essential oil is obtained from the needles of several pines, including *Pinus sylvestris* and *Abies sibirica*. It has a strong, resinous odour that is popular in refreshing toiletries and bath preparations. It is also useful for helping to relieve symptoms of the common cold. Pine has a stimulating effect on the circulation and is said to increase blood flow to the reproductive organs to increase desire for sex. It helps to restore positive feelings in those who have a negative self image, blame themselves or who feel helpless, unworthy or guilty. Pine essential oil combines well with lavender and lemon. Do not add more than two or three drops in a carrier oil blend added to a bath as it can cause skin irritation.

Rose

Rose is an essential oil obtained from two main types of rose, *Rosea centifolia* (French or Moroccan) and *rosa damascena* (Bulgarian). Oil of rose has variously been dedicated to Aphrodite, the Greek goddess of sexual love and beauty, and her Roman equivalent, Venus. Because the scent of rose is so sensual, the Romans scattered rose petals on bridal beds for the wedding night – a tradition now embodied in throwing confetti. Pure rose oil is, unfortunately, expensive as so many rose petals are needed to extract just a few grams of scent. It is so powerful however, that you only need one or two drops to use in sensual massage blends. Rose is one of the true prosexual aromatherapy oils. It especially appeals to female sexuality and is thought to stimulate secretion of pheromones. The aromatic substances found in the two different types of rose are slightly different, and the French or Moroccan rose oil (e.g. rose maroc) is reputed to have the more powerful aphrodisiac effect. It is especially useful for women who find it difficult to reach orgasm and whose low sex drive is linked with lack of self-confidence or with menstrual problems. It is also beneficial for men suffering from erection dysfunction. Rose is also soothing, calming and antidepressant and will help where low libido is associated with anxiety, insomnia and low mood. By warming the emotions, it also helps recovery after rejection, abuse or hurt while restoring the trust that makes love possible again. Rose essential oil combines well with most other oils, especially angelica, benzoin, bergamot, cardamom, cinnamon, clary-sage, coriander, cumin, fennel, geranium, ginger, jasmine, lemon, mace, neroli, nutmeg, patchouli, rosemary, rosewood, sandalwood, vanilla and ylang-ylang. Rose should be avoided during the first three months of pregnancy.

Rosemary

Rosemary is an essential oil extracted from the flowering tips and leaves of the popular culinary herb, *Rosemary officinalis*, which is native to the Mediterranean. It has a warm, penetrating aroma with a markedly stimulating and invigorating action. It also has a reputation for improving memory. Rosemary is useful where low sex drive is linked with physical exhaustion, confusion, mental fatigue and poor circulation. Rosemary is also useful for those with a poor sense of self-worth, lack of self-confidence and timidity. Rosemary essential oil combines well with bergamot, cardamom, cumin, fennel, geranium, lavender, lemon, juniper berry, mace, neroli, nutmeg, orange, patchouli, peppermint, rose, rosewood, sandalwood and ylang-ylang. Rosemary oil should not be used during pregnancy, or by people who have experienced epileptic fits. Rosemary should not be used if any homeopathic remedies are being taken as it will nullify their effects.

Rosewood

Rosewood is an essential oil derived from the wood of the rosewood tree, which is native to the Amazonian rainforest. It is a complex oil with floral, woody and spicy notes which may be used on its own or added to blends. It is used to boost immunity and to relieve headaches, especially where they occur with nausea. Rosewood oil has a calming, uplifting effect on the mood as well as an aphrodisiac action. It is especially useful where low sex drive is linked with stress, depression, fatigue and headache. Rosewood essential oil combines well with benzoin, bergamot, black pepper, cardamom, cinnamon, clary-sage, coriander, cumin, geranium, ginger, grapefruit, jasmine, lavender, lemon, mace, neroli, nutmeg, orange, patchouli, peppermint, rose, rosemary, sandalwood and vetiver.

Sandalwood

Sandalwood is an essential oil extracted from the heart of an evergreen tree, *Santalum album*, which is native to India. It is a powerful prosexual essential oil that has a strong, aromatic scent attractive to both men and women. It is sedative with both warming and strengthening properties that can reduce anxiety and lift self-confidence. Its sensual properties are partly due to its ability to relax, but some researchers believe it has an hormonal action in the body. It also seems to mimic or stimulate secretion of pheromones. Many people using it for other reasons later report a strong erotic effect, even when they had been unaware of its reputation as an aphrodisiac beforehand. Sandalwood is excellent for helping men to overcome impotence. Although it is thought of as a masculine aromatherapy oil, it also appeals to many women. Sandalwood is an excellent all-round aphrodisiac oil to boost sex drive. It is also helpful for those whose low libido is linked with agitation, anger, exhaustion, insomnia and obsessive traits. Sandalwood essential oil combines well with ambrette, angelica, benzoin, bergamot, black pepper, cardamom, clary-sage, cumin, fennel, geranium, ginger, jasmine, juniper berry, lemon, neroli, patchouli, rose, rosemary, rosewood, vetiver and ylang-ylang. Sandalwood and ylang-ylang together have a synergistic aphrodisiac effect.

(**NB** avoid essential oils of sandalwood originating from Australia or the West Indies, as these come from a totally different tree, *Eucarya spicata*, which does not have the same properties).

Vanilla

Vanilla is an oily resin that is mainly derived from the pods of a tropical, climbing orchid, *Vanilla planifolia*, which is native to Mexico, Central and South America. Some is also made from *Vanilla tahitensis* (native to the South Pacific) and *Vanilla pompona*. Fresh vanilla beans have no aroma, which only develops as a result of enzymatic actions during curing. The beans are sweated at night and exposed to sunlight during the day for up to two weeks until they become chocolate brown in colour. They are then dried for at least four months during which tiny crystals of vanillin form and become dissolved into the oily resin surrounding the seeds. Vanilla has a rich, intensely sweet and sensual aroma that is calming and helps to release pent up anger and frustration. Vanilla oil combines well with benzoin, bergamot, cinnamon, coriander, cumin, geranium, grapefruit, lavender, lemon, mace, neroli, nutmeg, orange, rose and ylang-ylang.

Vetiver

Vetiver (sometimes known as vetivert) is an essential oil derived from the roots of a fragrant grass, *Vetiveria zizanoides*, that is native to India. It has a smoky, earthy lemon aroma which adds a subtle note to blends. Vetiver is one of the true prosexual aromatherapy oils that stimulate secretion of pheromones and was used to anoint brides in ancient India. It has a profound, relaxing and calming effect and is traditionally referred to as the Oil of Tranquillity. It is a relaxing essential oil that is helpful for those whose sex drive is linked with stress, over-work, anxiety, low mood or insomnia. It is particularly useful for workaholics and perfectionists. Vetiver essential oil combines well with bergamot, clary-sage, geranium, ginger, jasmine, lavender, lemon, mace, neroli, nutmeg, orange, rosewood and sandalwood.

Ylang-ylang

Ylang-ylang is an essential oil derived from the petals of a tropical tree, *Canana odorata* which is native to the Philippines, Java, Sumatra and Madagascar. There are five grades of ylang-ylang, of which Extra Superior is just that but is unfortunately more expensive. The name ylang-ylang may mean 'flower of flowers' or may derive from the Philippine *alang-ilang*, meaning 'flowers that flutter in the breeze'. It has an exotic, voluptuous, spicy-sweet fragrance that is almost overpoweringly floral – like a cross between night-scented stock and almond blossom. Ylang-ylang is one of the true prosexual aromatherapy oils that stimulate secretion of pheromones. In Indonesia, the petals are spread on the honeymoon bed of newly married couples. It has the advantage of being cheaper than the other heady aphrodisiac oils, jasmine and rose, although some people dislike its intensity. When used in diluted form (one drop to one tablespoon carrier oil) those who dislike it may in fact find it exquisite. Ylang-ylang is both relaxing and uplifting and is helpful for impotence and total loss of sex drive in men or women. It is also helpful for those whose low sex drive is linked with stress, anxiety, over-breathing and trepidation which has swamped any sensual feelings. It also seems to have anti-epileptic properties. Ylang-ylang needs to be used sparingly as excess may have the opposite effect and reduce sex drive rather than increasing it. Ylang-ylang performs best mixed with other oils and combines well with angelica, benzoin, bergamot, black pepper, cardamom, cinnamon, clary-sage, coriander, cumin, geranium, ginger, grapefruit, jasmine, lavender, lemon, mace, neroli, nutmeg, orange, patchouli, rose, rosemary, sandalwood and vanilla. Ylang-ylang and sandalwood combined have a synergistic aphrodisiac effect.

How to use essential oils to boost your sex drive

Prosexual essential oils can be divided up depending on whether they have mainly masculine, feminine or hermaphrodite (male and female) qualities. As a general rule, oils classed as masculine tend to work better in men, while oils classed as feminine tend to work better in women. Essential oils classed as hermaphrodite are equally suitable for use by males or females.

Male essential oils with mainly masculine qualities include:	Female essential oils with mainly feminine qualities include:	Hermaphrodite essential oils that are both masculine and feminine at the same time include:
ambrette	angelica	benzoin
black pepper	coriander	bergamot
cardamom	fennel	clary-sage
cinnamon	grapefruit	geranium
cumin	lavender	jasmine
ginger	neroli	juniper berry
lemon	rose	mace
orange	rosemary	nutmeg
pine	vanilla	patchouli
rosewood	ylang-ylang	peppermint
sandalwood	pimento berry	
vetiver		

The best way to use aromatherapy oils is to select two, three or four compatible oils and blend them together. You should aim to include:

- At least one masculine and/or one hermaphrodite prosexual oil in a blend intended for use in a programme to boost low sex drive in a male (a feminine oil may also be included).
- At least one feminine and/or one hermaphrodite prosexual oil in a blend intended for use in a programme to boost low sex drive in a female (a masculine oil may also be included).

For general use, choose oils whose aroma you really like, or whose qualities you are instinctively drawn to. If you have a particular problem linked with your low sex drive, such as physical exhaustion, low mood, impotence or stress, include at least one oil in your blend that can help the problem according to the table overleaf:

	Physical tiredness or mental exhaustion	Low mood or mood swings	Stress-over work or insomnia	Menopause or period problems	Erectile problems	Postnatal	Prostate Problems
angelica	•	•		•			
benzoin	•	•	•		•		
bergamot		•	•				
black pepper	•				•		
cardamom	•						
clary-sage			•	•			
coriander		•	•				
fennel			•	•		•	
geranium		•	•	•			
ginger		•					
grapefruit		•	•				
jasmine		•	•		•	•	
juniper berry			•	•			•
lavender		•					
lemon	•	•					
neroli		•	•	•			
orange	•	•	•				
patchouli		•	•		•		
peppermint	•						
pimento berry							
pine	•	•			•		
rose		•	•	•	•		
rosemary	•				•		
rosewood	•	•	•				
sandalwood	•		•				
vanilla		•					
vetiver		•					
ylang ylang		•			•		

The essential oils should always be diluted in a carrier oil such as almond, jojoba or wheatgerm oil for massaging into the skin or adding to bath water. The dilution is important as oils that are too concentrated may have an adverse effect or cause skin irritation. Add a maximum total of one drop essential oil to each 2ml (24 drops) of carrier oil. Two teaspoons (10ml) of carrier oil should therefore contain no more than five drops of essential oil blend, while two tablespoons (30 ml) should contain no more than 15 drops of essential oil blend. Oils that are twice as dilute as this often suffice (i.e. only five drops essential oil blend per 20ml carrier oil). A 5ml medicinal teaspoon measure (or a 5ml syringe if you prefer) can be bought cheaply from a chemist to ensure accuracy as kitchen teaspoons tend to hold slightly less than 5ml.

When making up a blend, choose oils whose aromas you like – and preferably those that your lover likes, too. The following combinations are given as a suggestion of oils that go well together and which have particular sensual qualities. The balance in which they are blended together depends on you. If a blend suggests jasmine, orange and neroli, for example, and you adore neroli try adding three drops neroli, one drop orange and one drop jasmine to 10ml carrier oil. If you prefer jasmine, try mixing it in a blend of two drops jasmine, one drop neroli and two drops orange. Experiment until you find an aroma that you love – and which suits your mood best. If a blend isn't quite to your liking, add more drops of one or more of the oils – or introduce another that you feel is missing. Keep a note of the total number of drops used so that you can ensure it is correctly diluted by adding extra carrier oil. Altogether, every five drops of essential oil should be balanced with 10ml of carrier oil.

Then use the blend daily and you should expect to notice an effect within seven days. As your moods change, the effect of a particular blend – and your need for it – will wear off. You should then switch to another blend to gain the benefits of different oils.

Remember: add no more than a total of five drops essential oil to 5ml (1 medicinal teaspoon OR 60 drops) carrier oil except under the guidance of a qualified aromatherapist.

Cautions

- Do not take essential oils internally.
- Only use cinnamon essential oil to scent a room.
- Before using an essential oil blend on your skin, put a small amount on a patch of skin and leave it for at least an hour (patch test) to make sure you are not sensitive to it.
- Do not use essential oils if you are pregnant, or likely to be, except under specialist advice from a qualified aromatherapist.
- Do not use essential oils if you suffer from high blood pressure or epilepsy, except under specialist advice from a qualified aromatherapist.
- Keep essential oils away from the eyes.
- If you are taking homeopathic remedies, do not use peppermint, rosemary or lavender essential oils as these may neutralize the homeopathic effect.
- Essential oils are flammable, so do not put them on an open flame.

Try mixing one of the following blends that appeals to you:

Soothing & Sensual	Sensual Carnation	Orchid Nights
jasmine	black pepper	benzoin
orange	ylang-ylang	rose
neroli		vanilla

Erotic Spice	Spice Bouquet	Sugar & Spice
ginger	bergamot	lemon
mace	lemon	mace
pimento berry	nutmeg	nutmeg
	vetiver	vanilla

Turkish Delight	Total Surrender	Sensual
rose	lavender	clary-sage
lemon	geranium	rose
vanilla	ylang-ylang	ylang-ylang

Mystery of the East	Exotica	Ripe Dreams
rose	black pepper	clary-sage
sandalwood	neroli	geranium
patchouli	ylang-ylang	rose
		ylang-ylang

1001 Nights	Sensual Release	Men Only
clary-sage	clary-sage	ambrette
jasmine	geranium	black pepper
rose	lemon	lemon
		sandalwood

Passionate Tension	Warm Intentions	Building Tension
cumin	black pepper	ginger
rose	geranium	rose
jasmine	sandalwood	ylang-ylang
sandalwood	ylang-ylang	

Highly Responsive	Calm Before the Storm	Overdrive
angelica	bergamot	jasmine
clary-sage	rose	rose
sandalwood	rosewood	sandalwood
		ylang-ylang

Gingering Up	Renewed Interest	Warm & Sensual
benzoin	clary-sage	ambrette
ginger	jasmine	black pepper
sandalwood	ylang-ylang	geranium
		lemon

Heady Spice	SoftTouch	Women Only
benzoin	lavender	neroli
black pepper	lemon	vanilla
ylang-ylang	vanilla	ylang-ylang

Perfume

Add up to ten drops of your favourite sensual perfume – or a mix of up to three different oils – to 30 mls almond oil and use to dab behind your ears, in your cleavage, under your breasts and on your wrists.

Baths

Choose a single favourite sensual oil, or a blend of up to three. Add five drops of essential oil to a tablespoon of carrier oil (e.g. almond, avocado) and mix. Draw your bath so that it is comfortably hot, but don't add the aromatic oil mix until the taps are turned off. Close the bathroom door to keep in the vapours and soak for 15 – 20 minutes, preferably in candlelight.

Shower
Add eight drops of essential oil to a tablespoon (15ml) of carrier oil. After cleansing your body with soap or gel, rinse well then dip a wet sponge in the oil mix and use it to gently massage your whole body while under a warm jet spray.

Sauna
Add two drops of essential oil to 300ml (half a pint) of water and throw over the coals to evaporate.

Pot Pourri
Add a few drops of essential oils to a pot pourri mix to scent your bedroom. Refresh the scent regularly as it starts to fade.

Bed
Add two or three drops of a sensual essential oil to a tissue and allow to dry, before tucking under your pillow – and that of your partner.

Room Spray
Fill a small sprayer with 100ml water and add ten drops of sensual essential oils of your choice. Shake the sprayer well before using to perfume your bedroom. This mix can also be placed in special porous holders designed to sit over a radiator.

Ring Burner
An aromatherapy ring burner is designed to sit over a light bulb so the oils it contains are gently diffused by the heat energy of the bulb.

Scented Candles
Wax candles are available that are impregnated with a variety of essential oils, many of which are labelled as sensual. Use to

fragrance your bathroom and bedroom. Alternatively, add a few drops of your chosen essential oil to an oil-burning lamp for a similar effect.

How to give an aromatherapy massage

Giving and receiving an aromatherapy massage is a relaxing, pleasurable experience. Massage your partner for 30 minutes, then relax while the touch experience is returned. The following are the secrets of success.

Choose a firm surface such as lying on several towels spread on the floor.

Make sure the room is warm with gentle light and slow, relaxing background music.

Warm the massage oil or lotion by placing the bottle in a bowl of comfortably hot water. Alternatively, rub some oil in your hands to warm it before using.

Ask your partner to lie on his or her front, and cover them with a large bath towel. Expose the area you are working on and re-cover them before moving on.

Begin with long, flowing, simple strokes that follow body contours to warm the skin. Then, vary the pressure and length of stroke you use, keeping movements flowing and rhythmic with one hand in contact with their body at all times. Try alternating firm movements with feathery ones. If you find a muscle that seems knotted or tense, concentrate on that area with gentle kneading movements.

When you have finished massaging the back, ask your partner to turn over so you can work on their front. Stroke towards the heart and finish by holding your partner's feet for a few seconds as this helps to ground them.

Do not apply essential oils directly to the genitals, even when diluted, as they may be super-absorbed from the mucous membranes which do not have an outer, protective layer like skin elsewhere on the body.

12

The power of positive thought

Your mind is a powerful force you can harness and use to help boost a flagging sex drive. Transcendental meditation, for example, has been shown to lower levels of serotonin and prolactin and increase levels of DHEA, three factors that can individually increase a low sex drive, and which together produce a powerful effect.

Self-esteem

A positive self-esteem is essential for a healthy sex drive, yet for whatever reason, the most common self belief is 'I am not good enough'. It is easy to compare yourself unfavourably with others but it is also very destructive. Thoughts of being unworthy, unable to cope and being no good at sex tend to become self-fulfilling prophesies. In contrast, people who believe in themselves and are confident they can beat their low sex drive start to exude an aura that attracts positive reactions from others – a phenomenon usually described as luck.

Self-confidence can be enhanced by substituting positive, calming thoughts for those you find stressful and negative. 'I'm no good at sex' then becomes 'I AM good at sex'. If you say this frequently enough to yourself, the affirmation will automatically become part of your belief system and can have a profoundly calming effect in stressful times. Self-esteem can also be boosted through practising creative visualization.

Creative visualization

A useful pre-sleep exercise is creative visualization using a positive affirmation. Think of a positive phrase that is suitable for your particular situation. For example, imagine yourself as an accomplished lover with a healthy libido and boundless sexual energy. An appropriate affirmation is 'I am an attractive and sensual person', or 'I have a healthy sexual appetite'.

Every night, when lying in bed, imagine yourself feeling sexually aroused and initiating sex with your partner. Focus on how you will feel – the flushed skin, increased breathing rate, quickening pulse, and imagine the tingling and engorgement of your genitals. Concentrate on how you will approach your partner, how you will kiss and caress your lover, how you will feel as you become more and more aroused.

Imagine the sensual and erotic pleasures you will enjoy, then repeat your positive thought slowly and carefully to yourself.

Now touch the bed with the little finger of your left hand. Repeat the thought and touch the bed with the ring finger of your left hand while concentrating on the warm, sensual feeling of making love.

Now touch the bed with each individual finger (and thumb) of the left hand, before moving on to the right. Then reverse the process, touching the bed starting with the little finger of the right hand. By the time you have finished, you will have repeated your positive affirmation 20 times.

Repeat this procedure every night for a week, staying awake throughout the entire process. The following week, repeat the process but let yourself fall asleep when you are ready. The statement should now have become part of your normal thinking patterns.

You will be surprised what a difference this exercise in positive thought can make. Visualization is a powerful tool. If you say things to yourself like 'I can't see myself feeling sexy' or 'I can't picture myself wanting sex', then you can guarantee you will never achieve these goals. Good motivation involves thinking positive at every opportunity. You CAN regain your sex drive. You CAN feel sexually fulfilled, your love life CAN improve beyond all recognition. You just have to believe it is possible and you will find the way to make it happen. If you can picture the outcome you desire in your mind's eye, you have reinforced where you want to be – and will sub-consciously find it easier to get there.

Practising these positive thought exercises in a flotation tank will imprint your aims even more firmly in your mind.

Learning to love your body

Many people find sex awkward because they are ashamed of some aspect of their body. Here's an exercise in total honesty. Take off all your clothes in a warm room in front of a full-length mirror. Gentle, relaxing music will help as this exercise takes time to do properly.

Study your face, breasts, shoulders, waist, hips, bottom, thighs and ankles in a critical manner. Turn sideways onto the mirror and study your profile and rear view too. A triple mirror, or another long mirror placed at an angle makes this easier. Don't be afraid to be honest. It's the only way to galvanize yourself into action.

Write down a list of as many good points about yourself that you can find, e.g.:

- my lips are voluptuous
- my hair is thick and healthy
- my skin is soft and supple
- my abdomen is firm and flat
- my breasts are normal sized
- my penis is a good size

Now write down a list of all the negative things you thought about your body, e.g.:

- my lips are too thin
- my skin is dry
- my hair needs cutting
- my breasts are too large
- I'm beginning to get a paunch
- my penis is too small

Having studied your body, put on some loose, comfortable clothes and think about your personality and emotions. Write down all the positive things you can think of, e.g.:

- I am easy going
- I have a wicked sense of humour
- I get on well with people
- I am caring and loyal
- I am sensitive to other people's feelings

Finally, write down all the negative thoughts that come into your head, e.g.:

- my sex drive has vanished
- I don't feel sexy any more
- nobody could love me
- I'm no good in bed

Now look at the lists containing negative physical and emotional statements and turn these round into positive ones including any solutions. For example:

- *My lips look thin* becomes *I will learn make-up techniques to help my lips look thicker*.

- *My skin is dry* becomes *I can easily soften my skin with a body lotion and by treating myself to a salt scrub and aromatherapy massage.*
- *My hair needs cutting* becomes *I can easily improve the appearance of my hair by visiting the hairdresser.*
- *My breasts are too large* becomes *My breasts are a perfectly acceptable size.*
- *I'm beginning to develop a paunch* becomes *I can easily firm my abdomen through a combination of diet and exercise.*
- *My penis is too small* becomes *My penis is a perfectly normal size.*
- *My sex drive has vanished* becomes *I can easily help my sex drive to return by following a libido boosting programme.*
- *I don't feel sexy any more* becomes *I will feel sexy again by following a programme to boost my sex drive.*
- *Nobody could love me* becomes *I am easy to love.*
- *I'm no good in bed* becomes *I WILL become good in bed.*

The power of positive thought should not be underestimated. If you feel negative about aspects of your appearance or personality, your self esteem will suffer. Every day, read the lists of good things you wrote down about yourself and say the new positive statements out loud to reinforce your motivation to change. This will change your negative patterns of sub-conscious thought into positive ones that will help you shed your inhibitions and help you regain your sex drive.

Relaxation techniques

Relaxation techniques are essential to help reduce the stress that commonly leads to a lowered sex drive. A wide range of therapies are available, according to your mood and needs. Touch therapies such as acupressure, shiatsu, aromatherapy massage and reflexology are beneficial, while yoga and meditation will help you exert mind control over the physical responses of the body.

The art of meditation uses the power of concentration to direct all senses inwards. With practice, it is possible to maintain a level of spiritual awareness and tranquillity that transcends everyday life. It involves attaining complete relaxation by focusing thoughts on a single, abstract image or a low pitched hum called a mantra.

The Maharishi Mahesh Yogi developed Transcendental Meditation so it could be easily practised in the modern world. Transcendental Meditation uses a variety of Sanskrit mantras, each of which is a short word or phrase that is repeated silently in the mind to still the thoughts and approach a deeper level of consciousness. This helps to achieve a deep relaxation, which leads to enhanced inner joy, vitality, and creativity and can help you regain your sexual balance.

All the above relationship therapies are best started under the supervision of a teacher to ensure you do them correctly and obtain the most benefit. Here are some relaxation exercises you can use at home, however.

Whole body relaxation

Find somewhere quiet, warm and semi-dark to lie down. Remove your shoes and loosen tight clothing. Keep your eyes closed throughout the session.

First, lift your arms into the air, bending them at the elbow. Clench your fists hard and concentrate on the tension in these muscles. Breathe in deeply and slowly. As you breathe out, start to relax and let the tension in your arms drain away. Release your clenched fists and lower your arms gently beside you. Feel the tension flow out of them until your fingers start to tingle.

Now shrug your shoulders as high as you can. Feel the tension in your head, shoulders, neck and chest. Hold for a moment, then slowly let the tension flow away as you continue breathing gently and slowly.

Lift your head and push it forwards while tightening your facial muscles. Clench your teeth, frown and screw up your eyes. Hold this tension for a few seconds then gradually start to relax.

Continue in this way, working through the remaining muscles in your back, abdomen, buttocks and legs. Make sure tension does not creep back into the parts of your body you have already relaxed. A feeling of warmth should wash over the areas you have relaxed and your body should feel heavy relaxed. Breathe calmly and slowly as you feel all that tension drain away.

Imagine you are lying in a warm, sunny meadow with a stream bubbling gently beside you. Relax for at least twenty minutes, occasionally checking your body for tension.

Yoga breathing exercise: The triangle (Trikonasana)

Stand comfortably with your legs slightly more than a shoulder-width apart, and your feet facing forward.

Breathe in, and raise your right arm up alongside your left ear, stretching as high as possible. As part of the same movement, your right arm will follow over to the left, forming a graceful curve from your fingertips down to your right foot.

Breathe regularly and hold the position for at least 30 seconds, gradually increasing to one minute.

Make sure you keep looking forward, not down, that your knees and upper elbow are straight, and that your body and feet are not twisted.

Return to your original position as you inhale.

Repeat the exercise again moving to the right.

Mantra Meditation

Choose a warm, quiet room, draw the curtains and light a soft lamp or a few candles.

Take off your shoes and loosen your clothing. Sit or lie down in a comfortable position and concentrate on listening to a relaxation tape including natural Earth sounds such as running water, jungle noises, bird song or sea sounds. As you listen, repeat a personal calming mantra such as 'om' or 'calm' quietly to yourself. Tune into your breathing and feel the tension in your muscles slowly drift away. As you listen to the sound, imagine your body becomes increasingly weightless until you find yourself floating among clouds, bathed in healing sunlight. Repeat your mantra in your mind as you become more and more relaxed, so it becomes your cue to relaxation. In future times of stress, imagine the melodies of the relaxation tape in your mind and repeat your personal mantra to help stress slip away.

Activating the Tan Tien

A Chinese technique called the Inner Smile helps to activate the Tan Tien and may be helpful in boosting DHEA levels. It only takes a few minutes and brings rapid relaxation and rejuvenation to help leave stress behind.

Sit comfortably with your back straight and your arms relaxed at your side. Imagine something that makes you smile, and start to smile internally so it is only felt by you – it doesn't have to be visible. Let the smile shine out of your eyes and travel inwards to spread all over your body before concentrating just below your navel in the Tan Tien – the seat of your constitutional essence, or *Jing*. As the smile radiates within, it will generate a feeling of relaxation and calm. Once you feel relaxed, you can return to normal activity enriched by feelings of warmth, harmony and inner strength.

13

How to be your own sex therapist

Any frequency of making love is normal so long as both you and your partner are happy. Many couples share love, affection and a meaningful emotional relationship without a physically active sex life. Frequently however, particularly where sex has virtually petered out, one of the partners will be unhappy about the lack of a physical relationship while the other is unhappy about the sexual demands being place on them. In one survey for example, over a third of menopausal women felt that men wanted sex more often than they did themselves and that this was often a problem.

While it is best to seek professional advice where sexual problems are long-standing, it is possible to do some of the exercises suggested by psychosexual therapists on your own at home. If these do not help within a few weeks, it is important to seek professional advice.

Communication

Although it is difficult starting to talk about a sex problem, this is vital if a couple are to avoid drifting apart permanently. The discussion needs to be frank and open, not hidden behind gestures, inferences, veiled comments, jokes and put-downs. Set aside a time when neither of you are under pressure to be doing something else, and choose a neutral setting such as the lounge. Don't attempt this after you have just tried to make love or when either partner is feeling rejected, hurt or angry, or it may degenerate into a slanging match. Being your own sex therapist requires patience and perseverance as discussion needs to be honest, forthright and confronting if it is to be effective. The following guidelines are the secret of success:

- It is important to be clear in what you are saying, so think through beforehand what you want to say and how you are going to say it – this is very important when discussing emotionally-charged issues.
- Take it in turns to make a point and don't move on to the next issue until the first has been resolved.
- State your most important point first, and be concise without being simplistic or superficial.
- Be careful and sensitive in what you say.
- Don't talk AT your partner, give them a chance to respond.
- Don't express your feelings as a criticism or blame; use 'I' language – rather than saying *you* say *we,* e.g. 'I would prefer it if we…'
- Avoid generalizations e.g. 'You never kiss me' or 'You always do the same things'.
- Be positive – start off by saying what you like rather than what you don't like.
- Try not to criticize each other, but work together to find a way round any problems.
- Try not to feel defensive or aggressive.
- If your partner rejects a sexual activity that you want to try, remember they are not rejecting you – just the activity.
- Don't bring up old grievances that are not relevant to the point under discussion.
- Stick to the point and do not move on or get side-tracked until both of you are happy that it has been resolved.

- If you cannot agree on ways to approach a particular problem, you can mutually agree to put it to one side and come back to it later.
- If you are feeling hot under the collar, use a pre-arranged signal to take a break and cool off.
- If discussion fails, try writing down your feelings to each other in a letter instead ...

Sensate focusing

Psychosexual therapists often suggest a series of sexual exercises – known as sensate focusing, or pleasuring – for a couple to do at home. This involves setting aside time to explore each other's body, stroking, massaging and giving pleasure while communicating what you like and how it makes you feel.

You are encouraged to spend around an hour giving each other pleasure through massage (use aromatherapy oils for a sensual massage – *see Chapter 11*). Usually you start with non-sexual touching (non-genital sensate focusing) and avoid obviously erotic areas such as the breasts and genitals. Use all five senses – touch, taste, smell, sight and sound. Tell your partner what you like and how it could be better. After a while, swap places, and touch your partner in the way that gives you pleasure to see how they respond.

Once both partners are comfortable with this, you progress to the next stage of sexual touching, or Genital Sensate Focusing, in which erogenous zones can be touched as well. Oral sex and mutual masturbation is allowed, but penetrative sex is banned. This takes away the pressure to perform while helping to rekindle the flames. The object of genital sensate focussing is not orgasm, but to learn that arousal can be pleasurable in itself. After a while, swap places so you take it in turns to be active and passive.

It is important to make appreciate noises and smile when your partner does something you like, and to take their hand and guide them to areas you like to be touched. You can also show them how quickly, slowly, softly or firmly you like to be touched by placing your own fingers over theirs and literally showing them what to do.

Eventually, sometimes after more than 20 sessions lasting an hour each, the couple will feel ready to try penetration – but without movement (i.e. no thrusting). This exercise aims to prove that orgasm is not essential with penetration. After you are both aroused, the female guides the man inside her, and is allowed to contract her pelvic floor muscles but nothing else. The man is banned from thrusting. You should remain coupled but still for several minutes, and disengage before orgasm. You can repeat penetration as often as you wish, as long as there is no movement once inside. This helps to prolong the phase of giving one another pleasure. Orgasm may then be reached through mutual masturbation but without penetration.

Finally, penetration with movement is allowed. After the penis is inside her, only the woman is allowed to move at first. Then she should lie still and the man is allowed to make slow, gentle movements. Continue taking turns before withdrawing every so often and continuing to caress and stroke each other. After several session, you are allowed to reach climax during penetrative sex with movement.

Sensate focusing is surprisingly successful as both partners remain in control at all times within the strict guidelines.

Erogenous zones

To give and receive pleasure during sensate focussing, you need to know where to find the erogenous zones. Erogenous zones are important as they provide a short cut to arousal when making love. The erogenous zones are sensitive areas of skin that are covered with an increased number of nerve endings. When these areas are stimulated in the right way, they can trigger sensual feelings and sexual arousal. Your major erogenous zones include all the obvious sites. In females, these are the lips, buttocks, breasts, nipples and external genitals including the clitoris and vaginal entrance. In men, the major zones are the lips, nipples, penis and scrotum.

Everyone also has secondary erogenous zones. These include the back of the neck, the eyelids, ears and earlobes plus the soft skin at the top of the inner thighs. Most people are also very sensitive around the anus, but be careful. Although this sensation is pleasurable for some, others find it distinctly uncomfortable.

During foreplay, the erogenous zones can be stimulated by gentle stroking, licking, blowing or nibbling. As the secondary erogenous zones vary from person to person, gently blowing on the back of the neck is a turn-on for some, whilst others find licking behind the knees, having their toes sucked or their earlobes nibbled more erotic.

Working out where your own zones are – and finding those of your partner – is half the fun of making love.

Once you have discovered where your partner's erogenous zones are, you can try more advanced techniques for stimulating them. Use a feather to make long, soft, tickly sweeps down the insides of his thighs, or use a vibrator on the backs of the knees. Some men adore having their scrotum or the back of their neck stimulated alternately with warm and then icy cold water.

Finding the G-spot

The G-spot is a controversial erogenous zone that is only present in women. It is named after the person who first described it, Ernst Graffenberg, and is said to be a button-like area of tissue on the front wall of the vagina that swells up during sexual stimulation. When it is stimulated and gently pressed, it is said to lead to instant orgasm that is much stronger than a clitoral orgasm.

Pressing the G-spot button supposedly also stimulates secretion of a mysterious fluid. This fluid apparently comes out at quite a force, similar to a male ejaculation. Unfortunately, no anatomists or physiologists have been able to find any tissue that fits this description and the existence of the G-spot is still in hot dispute.

The upper third of the vagina is sensitive to stretch and does swell and balloon outwards quite considerably. This produces an intense desire for penetration. During sexual excitement, the vaginal tissues become quite engorged as local blood vessels dilate. It's possible that in some women, this tissue swelling produces a button-like area at the front of the vagina.

This engorgement forces fluid under pressure out of the blood vessels into surrounding tissues. Some women become so engorged and produce so much lubrication, that it may seem as if they are leaking fluid during orgasm. Research using ultra-sound probes in the vagina has shed new light on what happens during sexual intercourse. The thrusting action of the penis produces quite remarkable stretching and thinning of the front wall of the vagina which means that some women leak urine during sex.

Because of where it is, it is virtually impossible for a woman to find her own G-spot. But there's nothing to stop you and your partner looking for it together as part of your love-making technique. Who knows – you might succeed in finding it! With his palm upwards, your partner should insert his lubricated index finger two to three inches into your vagina. He should then make a beckoning gesture with his finger to bring the fingertip against the vaginal front wall. He should be able to feel the underlying hardness of your pubic bone. He should then press his finger tip firmly up against this bone and move his fingertip round and round in a small circle. When you suddenly feel a strange, pleasant sensation, you've got it!

Don't be too disappointed if it remains elusive. Millions of women have sought their G-spot and failed.

Pelvic floor exercises

Pelvic floor exercises are beneficial for both men and women. By toning up the pelvic area, you can intensify sensations when making love and help to boost your sex drive.

Women

The vagina is surrounded by pelvic floor muscles that grip the penis when making love. Research suggests that as many as 40% of women lack normal tone in their pelvic floor muscles. This can interfere with sexual pleasure and lead to urinary leakage known as stress incontinence. As many as 1 in 4 women suffer at some time during their life – including in their 20s and 30s – usually as a result of childbirth.

Health specialists recommend that every women aged 16 and over should practise pelvic floor exercises for ten minutes a day. By toning up your pelvic muscles – especially those making up your pelvic floor – you can tighten your vaginal muscles and strengthen contractions during climax. Improving the strength and flexibility of these muscles will also improve your range of movement and make sexual positions such as squatting on top of your partner, or wrapping your legs round him easier and more comfortable. You will also be able to grip your partner more firmly when he is inside you, which will increase sexual pleasure for both of you. As well as improving your sex life, and helping you to have more and better orgasms, tightening up loose pelvic tissues will help to prevent future urinary leakage through stress incontinence.

Increasing your level of general exercise will help too. Research shows that pelvic floor muscles can also be strengthened beneficially by swimming, yoga, walking and other keep fit activities.

For general toning up of pelvic muscles and to reduce congestion, try the following three exercises. They are best performed after a bath or shower when you are warm and relaxed.

- Stand with your feet apart and your knees slightly bent.
  Place your hands on your hips, jut your bottom out and
  rotate your pelvis slowly in a clockwise direction. Continue
  rotating your pelvis round to form a complete circle that is
  as wide as possible. Continue these pelvic gyrations for 1–2
  minutes, then gyrate your pelvis round in an anti-clockwise
  direction for another 1–2 minutes.
- Pull up the front and back passages tightly as if trying to
  stop the bowels from opening. Hold tight for a count of four
  and repeat this every quarter of an hour.
- When on the loo, practise stopping the flow of urine mid-
  stream. Initially this will be difficult but when it becomes
  easy, do this at least once a day. When you've learned to
  identify which muscles are squeezed during this action, you
  can then practise clenching them several times a day even
  when not urinating. Don't overdo it however – new research
  suggests that repeatedly stopping urination may aggravate
  urinary problems. Use this exercise only to help identify
  the muscles you should be squeezing.
- Stand with your feet wide apart, and squat right down so
  your knees are bent and your bottom is just off the floor.
  Rest your fingers or palms on the floor between your feet,
  and let your buttocks drop down as far as possible. Breathe
  in deeply, then breathe out, letting your anus and pelvic floor
  muscles relax. Then breathe in four or five short breaths
  without exhaling in between. With each breath in, draw up
  and tighten your pelvic floor muscles as if pulling up your
  vagina step by step. Then breathe out five times slowly
  (without inhaling in between) and release your pelvic floor
  muscles in short steps. Repeat ten times.
- Women who don't mind touching themselves intimately can
  do an additional pelvic floor exercise. Insert two fingers inside

the vagina and try to squeeze them by contracting and
tightening your vaginal muscles. Once you are adept at it, you
can practise squeezing your partner when making love, too.

● Weighted cones (Aquaflex) to tighten and tone vaginal
muscles are also available. Cones make pelvic floor exercises
more effective. These vaginal weights are inserted like a
tampon for up to 10 minutes twice a day (see Resources).

Men

Men can also tone up their pelvic floor muscles to release tension
and congestion and to improve the flow of sexual energy. These
exercises are best performed after a bath or shower when you are
warm and relaxed.

The easiest way to identify the pelvic floor muscles is to start urinating, then concentrate on stopping the flow mid stream. Practise
this every time you visit the bathroom until you are able to accu-
rately squeeze these muscles at will and can start exercising them
regularly. Start with ten quick squeezes, holding each one for the
count of three. Repeat two or three times a day. Build up to 20 quick
squeezes at a time, holding each for the count of three. After around
a month, add in five long, slow squeezes after your 20 quick
squeezes. Squeeze in to a count of ten, then hold for a count of ten.
When you are comfortable with these, build up to ten long, slow
squeezes after each series of 20 quick squeezes.

The following exercises will also help to relieve pelvic tension.

● Stand with your feet apart and your knees slightly bent. Hold
your arms by your side with your palms facing forwards.
Breathe in deeply and pull your pelvis back. As you breathe
out, let your pelvis rock forward and arms, hands and
genitals move upwards. Repeat in a smooth, continuous
motion for 2 minutes.

- Stand with your feet apart and your knees slightly bent. Place your hands on your hips, jut your bottom out and rotate your pelvis slowly in a clockwise direction. Continue rotating your pelvis round to form a complete circle that is as wide as possible. Continue for 1 minute, then switch to a similar, anti-clockwise direction for another 1 minute.

- Lie on the ground, pushing the small of your back down so that it touches the floor, with knees bent, soles flat on the floor, and arms palm-down by your side. As you breathe out, roll your bottom upwards so it lifts off the floor, clenching your buttocks and inner thigh muscles. As you breathe out, roll your bottom down to the floor again and relax your clenched muscles. Repeat five to ten times.

- The Chinese believe that squeezing the prostate gland increases secretion of sex hormones and boosts libido. You can do this while sitting, standing or lying, whichever you prefer. Squeeze your anal muscles together tightly and hold for as long as is comfortable. Relax for a minute or two then repeat as many times as is comfortable.

Bridge Manoeuvre

Some women have a low sex drive because they are unable to achieve orgasm during penetrative sex. It is important to realize that this is quite common – in fact it could almost be classed as normal for the female not to achieve orgasm during the thrusting action of intercourse itself. Most women require direct clitoral stimulation plus an emotional input to reach climax.

A technique called the bridge manoeuvre can help to rekindle sexual interest during sex itself. Quite simply, the male masturbates the female until she is on the point of climax, then quickly inserts his penis to trigger her orgasm.

Seeking further help

Couples with profound sexual problems will benefit from referral to a psychosexual or relationship counsellor. Unlike relatives and friends, a professional therapist will provide a sympathetic listening ear without judgement, prejudice or jumping in with their own thoughts and experiences.

Different types of counselling offer different approaches to the problem. The following overview looks at the types of counselling that can help different situations.

Counselling

Standard counselling is designed to help you overcome a particular problem related to your low sex drive. It aims to let you see things in a new light so you can understand your emotions better. Counsellors will help you explore your options, reach your own solutions and act on them – they don't usually advise you what to do. Counselling is helpful if you:

- need help overcoming a specific problem such as alcohol abuse or an extremely stressful situation
- need help untangling the web of emotions surrounding a particular situation
- are in a crisis
- feel anxious or depressed.

Psychotherapy

Psychotherapy involves a more in-depth, longer course of treatment than counselling. It is based on the belief that what happened to you as a child (e.g.your parents expectations of you, your place in the family pecking order, your emotional interactions with family and schoolfriends) have a major effect on your personality and behaviour patterns in adulthood. Psychotherapy probes your subconscious feelings to explore your memories, dreams, fears, desires and fantasies. Different therapists use different techniques, which may involve:

- free association (reporting everything that comes into your head while you are relaxed, no matter how trivial, unpleasant or embarrassing it may seem)
- transference (a process in which you transfer your emotions for other people onto the therapist, so you subconsciously reveal your anger, hurt or resentment)
- dream interpretation or
- hypnotherapy.

Psychotherapy is helpful if you:

- feel stuck in a rut
- have a long-standing, deep-seated problem linked with your low libido
- would like to feel more confident
- feel cut off from your emotions
- want to know yourself better
- would like to change the way you behave
- suffer from anxiety, depression, an obsessive compulsive disorder, a phobia, addiction or eating problem.

Person-centred psychotherapy

This therapy helps you to tune in to your own untapped, internal resources so you develop a more positive self-image and reach self-fulfillment. The therapist generates an unconditional, positive warmth towards you, together with an empathy and genuineness that accepts you as you are. Therapy can help you become more spontaneous, less introverted and more in control as a result of feeling understood and valued by the therapist.

Person-centred psychotherapy is helpful if you:

- often feel worthless or unloved
- would value a close, caring friendship where you can talk person-to-person
- find it difficult to accept compliments
- feel little satisfaction with your life
- feel you need space to grow
- feel you have hidden resources
- find it difficult to talk about your feelings.

Art psychotherapy

Art psychotherapy helps you explore your feelings and develop a deeper self-awareness by expressing yourself in a non-verbal way. This may take the form of painting, drawing or modelling (art therapy); singing or playing musical instruments (music therapy); dancing (dance movement therapy) or acting (drama therapy). Talent is not important – the therapist analyzes how you express yourself to reveal the inner conflicts preventing you from leading a fulfilling life.

Art psychotherapy is helpful if you:

- find it difficult to express how you feel in words alone
- want to develop a strong sense of yourself without the need for too much conventional talk counselling.

Transactional analysis therapy

Transactional analysis centres around the belief that everyone has three basic personality traits: parent, adult and child. One of these emotional states is to the fore at any one time, and problems arise when you adopt one that is inappropriate for a particular situation. The therapist helps you understand which personality trait is active at any one time so you can understand and change any harmful patterns.

Transactional analysis therapy is helpful if you:

- lead a life that is all work and no play
- are continually seeking excitement and failing to find satisfaction
- are excessively clinging
- are very strict and authoritarian
- hate or can't cope with responsibility.

Behaviour therapy

Behavioural therapy helps you overcome harmful and negative behaviour patterns. It involves relaxation techniques and developing positive thoughts in place of negative ones. Cognitive therapy is similar to behaviour therapy but delves deeper and explores some of the reasons why a particular problem has arisen.

Psychosexual therapy is a form of behaviour therapy in which a couple are counseled about relationship and sexual difficulties. Psychosexual therapy may involve sensate focusing techniques as described above. You may also be encouraged to identify and resolve emotional conflicts – past and present – that may be affecting your sex drive.

Psychosexual therapy is very helpful for treating:

- low sex drive
- premature or retarded ejaculation
- some forms of impotence
- pain and tenseness during sex
- difficulty reaching orgasm.

How to find a qualified counsellor

As counselling services are unregulated, anyone can call themselves a psychologist, counsellor or psychotherapist. It is important to ensure that the therapist you consult is properly trained and experienced, in which case they will usually be a member of a professional body that holds a register of qualified practitioners. Avoid any so-called therapist who offers to act as a sex surrogate, wants to observe sexual activities or suggests you engage in sex exercises in their presence. It is acceptable for a medically qualified sex therapist to examine you where an anatomical abnormality is suspected, however.

14

Prescription drugs to boost your sex drive

While many prescription drugs have an adverse effect on sexuality, a few are able to increase sex drive. These drugs are only touched on here for completeness.

NB no drugs should be used during pregnancy or when breast-feeding.

Deprenyl

Deprenyl (also known as selegiline) is a drug used to treat Parkinson's disease. As well as improving this condition, it also has a beneficial effect on memory, attention span and energy levels and is now also used successfully in some people with Alzheimer's disease. One of the most noticeable side effects is increased interest in sex in those taking it – especially in men aged 50 and over.

Deprenyl/selegiline is chemically related to phenylethylamine (PEA) the stimulant found in chocolate which helps to boost mood and which is also released in the brain during orgasm and when falling in love. Deprenyl/selegiline is thought to have several effects on the brain. The most understood effect is to block the activity of an enzyme (monoamine oxidase-B or MAO-B) that breaks down certain nerve communication chemicals, including dopamine. These means that dopamine levels remain higher and once released, it has an effect for longer. Deprenyl/selegiline particularly increases dopamine levels in a part of the brain called the substantia nigra, that regulates movement control (which goes awry in Parkinson's disease), immune function, motivation and sex drive.

With increasing age, brain levels of MAO-B increase and levels of dopamine start to fall from around the age of 40 to 45. As dopamine levels fall, so does interest in sex. Deprenyl/selegiline seems to overcome this, increases libido and makes orgasm easier to achieve. This may lead to an unwanted side effect of producing premature ejaculation. Other drugs which also block a similar enzyme, MAO-A, increase levels of several other neurotransmitters and can cause side effects of anxiety and high blood pressure, particularly after eating foods rich in tyramine, such as cheese and Chianti wine.

Deprenyl/selegiline is also being promoted as a miracle, longevity drug as it has been shown to extend maximum life-span in experimental animals by up to 40%. This may be because the ageing process is regulated in the substantia nigra or may be linked to the drug's antioxidant action in the brain.

Deprenyl/selegiline appears to have few side effects in the low doses prescribed to boost sex drive. Few doctors in the UK are likely to prescribe it for this indication, although it is popular in some countries such as the US.

Dose

It is usually given as liquid drops with the dose varying according to age. Initial starting dose (for the prosexual effect) is 1mg daily from the age of 35, increasing by 1mg per day every five years, so that by the age of 80 years, 10mg daily is taken (5mg twice daily). Larger starting doses are used for treating Parkinsonism.

Adverse reactions that have been reported at higher doses include low blood pressure, nausea, vomiting, confusion, agitation, dry mouth, sleep disturbances, difficulty passing water and skin rashes.

Excess dopamine has also been linked with the development of psychotic behaviour, such as schizophrenia.

Should only be used under medical supervision.

Bromocriptine

Bromocriptine is a drug that, like deprenyl/selegiline, increases levels of dopamine in the brain and is used to help treat Parkinson's disease. Bromocriptine also has a powerful ability to lower raised levels of prolactin hormone and is used to help treat hyperprolactinaemia (e.g. due to a pituitary tumour) and to suppress or prevent lactation. Some evidence also suggests that bromocriptine can increase testosterone levels where these are low.

Bromocriptine is available on prescription in most countries and can be used to treat low sex drive where this is linked with hyperprolactinaemia.

Possible side effects include nausea, vomiting, constipation, headache, dizziness, low blood pressure, drowsiness and Raynaud's syndrome. In high doses may cause confusion hallucinations, dry mouth, leg cramps, pleural effusions or retroperitoneal fibrosis. Should only be used under medical supervision.

Viagra

Viagra (Sildenafil) is an effective drug treatment for treating male impotence. It is available on prescription in some countries such as the US and the UK, and awaiting a product licence for marketing in others. Its main action is to selectively inhibit Type 5 phosphodiesterase receptors in the penis to trigger erection. This relaxes smooth muscle fibres in the penis and its blood supply so that more blood arrives into the area and erection results. Unfortunately, there is currently little evidence that Viagra will boost a flagging sex drive in men who are not impotent, or in women, although small trials are underway to investigate this possibility. *For more information, see Chapter 4.*

Should only be used under medical supervision.

Yohimbine hydrochloride

Yohimbine hydrochloride is a chemical derived from a tree (Pausinystalia yohimbe or Corynanthe yohimbe) native to West Africa. It is available on prescription in some countries to treat male impotence at doses of around 5mg to 42mg daily (*for more information see pages 171–2*).

Should only be used under medical supervision.

Testosterone and oestrogen replacement therapy

A low sex drive linked with the female menopause or low levels of testosterone hormone in the male may be helped by hormone replacement therapy (*for further details see Chapter 8*).

Should only be used under medical supervision.

Further reading: *Better Sex Through Chemistry*, by John Morgenthaler & Dan Joy (*see Resources section*).

15

Boost your sex drive:
individually tailored plans

Follow the dietary and lifestyle advice given below, while at the same time following one of the libido enhancing plans at the end of this chapter.

Six male plans and six female plans based on a 12-week programme are included, designed to help:

1. Healthy men under 45 whose low sex drive is not linked with any particular condition
2. Men under 45 whose low sex drive is linked with erectile dysfunction
3. Men of any age whose low sex drive is linked with overwork, exhaustion or stress
4. Healthy men over 45 with no prostate symptoms or erectile dysfunction
5. Men over 45 with prostate symptoms
6. Men over 45 with erectile dysfunction

1. Younger women with a low sex drive
2. Women whose low sex drive is linked with premenstrual syndrome
3. Women who have had a baby and are breastfeeding
4. Women who have had a baby but are not breastfeeding
5. Mature women during and after the menopause
6. Non-oestrogenic plan for women advised to avoid oestrogenic supplements (e.g. because of a potentially oestrogen-sensitive condition such as breast cancer).

Women under stress should follow the plan for healthy women of the appropriate age group.

Lifestyle changes

- Follow a healthy, wholefood, organic diet with at least one vegetarian day per week.
- Avoid overwork and excess stress. Try to find time for relaxation techniques such as breathing exercises, meditation and yoga.
- Get plenty of sleep.
- Take regular exercise to boost your DHEA levels.
- Lose excess weight.
- Try to cut out alcohol altogether for at least a month, or reduce your intake to no more than one or two units per day. If you do not wish to give up alcohol completely, try to have at least one alcohol-free day per week.
- If you smoke, try to stop: chemicals in cigarette smoke lower sex hormone levels.
- Check that a low sex drive is not an unwanted side effect of any tablets you are taking.
- Naturopaths advise cold showers and baths to invigorate and increase both the metabolic rate and production of testosterone.

Look after your relationship:

- Talk about problems openly.
- Find time to talk.
- Don't neglect family and friends because of work.
- Show affection for each other.
- Make sure you are still friends.

Read the chapters on positive thought and how to be your own sex counsellor.

Plan which prosexual supplements you will take to boost your sex drive, and buy them from a health food shop or via mail order (*see Resources for details*).

Select the sensual aromatherapy oils whose scent appeals to you most.

Health and relaxation

- Do some pelvic floor exercises to tone up your genital area (see Chapter 14).
- Go for a brisk walk or take part in another, invigorating form of exercise for half an hour a day.
- Relax in a luxury bubble bath (scented with your chosen aromatherapy oils).
- Pursuade your partner to give you an aromatherapy massage (*see Chapter 11*).
- Write down ten things you like about yourself.
- Make an appointment to have a hair cut, facial, manicure, pedicure, join a gym – anything that will raise your self-confidence, elevate your self esteem and improve your health or appearance.
- Think positive. This is the first day of the rest of your life. Make regaining your sex drive one of your main priorities.

Men: Boost your sex drive

- Follow the diet and lifestyle plan at the beginning of this chapter, ensuring you have a good intake of vitamins and minerals.
- Consider using a pheromone preparation (see Chapter 5).
- If you wish to try aromatherapy, select essential oils from the charts and blends given in Chapter 11. If you are also taking homeopathic remedies, do not use peppermint, rosemary or lavender essential oils as these may neutralize the homeopathic effect.

Follow one of six tailored programmes below, designed to suit the needs of:

1. Healthy men under 45 whose low sex drive is not linked with any particular condition.
2. Men under 45 whose low sex drive is linked with erectile dysfunction.
3. Men of any age whose low sex drive is linked with overwork, exhaustion or stress.
4. Healthy men over 45 with no prostate symptoms or erectile dysfunction.
5. Men over 45 with prostate symptoms.
6. Men over 45 with erectile dysfunction.

Some supplements are available in health food stores or chemists, others by mail order (*see Resources*).

1. Healthy under 45's plan

Basic Supplements to take throughout the programme:

- A multivitamin and mineral supplement providing around 100% of the recommended daily amount (RDA) of as many micronutrients as possible, plus important trace elements such as boron, chromium, copper and molybdenum (e.g. Centrum). Blue-green algae is a suitable alternative if you prefer.

- Evening primrose oil (1000mg per day) to provide the essential fatty acids, needed for synthesis and balance of sex hormones.
- Consider taking Co-enzyme Q10 if you feel lacking in energy.

Weeks 1 – 6: Viryl-forte (Larkhall Green Farm, *see Resources*).

Weeks 7 – 12: If you have started to notice a benefit, continue with the supplements you are taking.

If you have not noticed a benefit, add in, or switch to, one or more of the following supplements having first read about them in the relevant chapter to see which would suit you best:

- catuaba: 1gm twice daily
- Libido (chicken egg extracts): 6 capsules morning and evening for one week, then 2 capsules morning and evening thereafter
- Touchfire His drops for men (Muira puama, catuaba, damiana, sarsaparilla and nettle root): 30 – 40 drops in water, twice a day
- L-arginine: 150mg to 3g daily, ideally one hour before sex
- Korean ginseng: 600mg daily
- DHEA (if aged over 40) or wild yam complexes designed to entrance natural DHEA production
- Tribulus terrestris: 250mg daily
- fo-ti: 5g daily
- ashwagandha: 150 – 300 mg
- Intra (Healthcare International): 30ml daily
- bee pollen: 250mg – 2g daily

- Love Life: 3 tablets twice a day
- Male Plus: 30 – 40 drops in water, twice a day

If you wish to use a homeopathic remedy, select one of the following, having first read Chapter 10: arsenicum album; agnus castus; Amphosca for Men, arsenicum album; baryta carbonica; conium maculatum; cuprum metallicum; graphites; Love Life; moschus moschiferus; nux vomica; phosphoricum acidum; sulphur; homeopathic hormones (e.g. testosterone, DHEA) may be prescribed by a qualified practitioner.

If at the end of the programme, there is no significant improvement in your sex drive, consult your doctor in case you need further investigations (e.g. prolactin or other hormone measurements) and treatment.

2. Under 45's erectile dysfunction plan
Basic Supplements to take throughout the programme:

- A multivitamin and mineral supplement providing around 100% of the recommended daily amount (RDA) of as many micronutrients as possible, plus important trace elements such as boron, chromium, copper and molybdenum (e.g. Centrum). Blue-green algae is a suitable alternative if you prefer.
- Evening primrose oil (1000mg per day) to provide the essential fatty acids, needed for synthesis and balance of sex hormones.
- Ginkgo biloba: Extracts standardized for at least 24% ginkolides: 40 – 60mg 2 to 3 times a day (take a minimum of 120mg daily).
- Consider taking Co-enzyme Q10 if you feel lacking in energy.

Weeks 1 – 6: catuaba (Rio Trading): 1g twice a day

Weeks 7 – 12: If you have started to notice a benefit, continue with the supplements you are taking.

If you have not noticed a benefit, add in, or switch to, one or more of the following supplements having first read about them in the relevant chapter to see which would suit you best:

- Touchfire His drops for men: (muira puama, catuaba, damiana, sarsaparilla and nettle root) 30 to 40 drops in water, twice a day
- Muira puama 1 – 1.5g daily for two weeks
- Libido (chicken egg extracts): 6 capsules morning and evening for one week, then 2 capsules morning and evening thereafter
- Korean ginseng 600mg daily for 6 weeks
- L-arginine 150mg to 3g daily, ideally one hour before sex
- DHEA (if aged over 40) or wild yam complexes designed to enhance natural DHEA production
- Tribulus terrestris: 250mg daily
- fo-ti 5g daily
- ginger: 250mg two to four times
- sarsaparilla: 250mg three times a day
- ashwagandha: 150 – 300 mg
- bee pollen: 250mg – 2g daily
- Love Life: 3 tablets twice a day
- Male Plus: 30 – 40 drops in water, twice a day

If you wish to use a homeopathic remedy, select one of the following, having first read Chapter 10: Amphosca for Men; arsenicum album; Bach Rescue Remedy; baryta carbonica; conium maculatum; graphites; Love Life; lycopodium; plumbum metallicum; sulphur; homeopathic hormones (e.g. testosterone, DHEA) may be prescribed by a qualified practitioner.

If at the end of the programme, there is no significant improvement in your sex drive, consult your doctor in case you need further investigations (e.g. prolactin or other hormone measurements) and treatment.

3. Men of any age whose low sex drive is linked with overwork, exhaustion or stress

Basic Supplements to take throughout the programme:

- A multivitamin and mineral supplement providing around 100% of the recommended daily amount (RDA) of as many micronutrients as possible, plus important trace elements such as boron, chromium, copper and molybdenum (e.g. Centrum). Blue-green algae is a suitable alternative if you prefer.
- Evening primrose oil (1000mg per day) to provide the essential fatty acid, needed for synthesis and balance of sex hormones.
- Korean ginseng 600mg daily: four weeks on, four weeks off regime. If you find this too stimulating, switch to Siberian ginseng (eleutherococcus senticosus) 1g twice a day for 12 weeks.
- Consider taking Co-enzyme Q10 (90mg daily) for lack of energy.
- Consider taking Milk Thistle if your intake of alcohol is high.

Weeks 1 – 6: Libido (chicken egg extracts): 6 capsules morning and evening for one week, then 2 capsules morning and evening thereafter.

Weeks 7 – 12: If you have started to notice a benefit, continue with the supplements you are taking.

If you have not noticed a benefit, add in, or switch to, one or more of the following supplements having first read about them in the relevant chapter to see which would suit you best:

- Tribulus terrestris 250mg daily
- ashwagandha: 150 – 300 mg
- catuaba: 1gm twice daily
- Touchfire His drops for men: (muira puama, catuaba, damiana, sarsaparilla and nettle root) 30 to 40 drops in water, twice a day
- Muira puama 1 – 1.5g daily for two weeks
- Ginkgo biloba: Extracts standardized for at least 24% ginkolides: 40 – 60mg 2 to 3 times a day (take a minimum of 120mg daily)
- gotu kola: 60 – 120mg daily
- guarana 1g daily
- reishi: 500mg two to three times daily
- schisandra: 250mg – 500mg once to three times daily
- sarsaparilla: 250mg three times a day
- Intra (Healthcare International) 30ml daily
- oats (oatstraw): 3ml tincture three times a day
- bee pollen: 250mg – 2g daily
- Love Life: 3 tablets twice a day
- Male Plus: 30 – 40 drops in water, twice a day

If you wish to use a homeopathic remedy, select one of the following, having first read Chapter 10: agnus castus; Amphosca for Men; arsenicum album; Bach Rescue Remedy; baryta carbonica; calcarea carbonica; cuprum metallicum; gelsemium sempervirens; Love Life; moschus moschiferus; nux vomica; phosphoricum acidum.

If at the end of the programme, there is no significant improvement in your sex drive, consult your doctor in case you need further investigations (e.g. prolactin or other hormone measurements) and treatment.

4. Healthy over–45's plan

Basic supplements to take throughout the programme:

- Evening primrose oil (1000mg per day) to provide the essential fatty acids, needed for synthesis and balance of sex hormones.
- Consider taking Co-enzyme Q10 if you feel lacking in energy.

Weeks 1 – 6: Kordel's Zest for Men: One tablet daily (contains vitamins, minerals, damiana, Siberian ginseng, oyster extract, sarsaparilla, saw palmetto and cayenne).

Weeks 7 – 12: If you have started to notice a benefit, continue with the supplements you are taking.

If you have not noticed a benefit, add in one, or switch to, or more of the following supplements having first read about them in the relevant chapter to see which would suit you best:

- catuaba: 1gm twice daily
- Libido (chicken egg extracts): 6 capsules morning and evening for one week, then 2 capsules morning and evening thereafter
- Touchfire His drops for men: (Muira puama, catuaba, damiana, sarsaparilla and nettle root) 30 to 40 drops in water twice a day
- L-arginine: 150mg to 3g daily, ideally one hour before sex
- Korean ginseng: 600mg daily
- DHEA or wild yam complexes designed to enhance natural DHEA production
- saw palmetto fruit extracts: 150mg – 3g daily in divided doses; products standardized for 85% – 95% fat-soluble sterols: 320mg daily
- Tribulus terrestris: 250mg daily
- fo-ti: 5g daily

- ashwagandha: 150 – 300 mg
- Intra (Healthcare International) 30ml daily
- bee pollen: 250mg – 2g daily
- Love Life: 3 tablets twice a day
- Male Plus: 30 – 40 drops in water, twice a day

If you wish to use a homeopathic remedy, select one of the following, having first read Chapter 10: agnus castus; Amphosca for Men, arsenicum album, baryta carbonica; conium maculatum; cuprum metallicum; graphites; Love Life; moschus moschiferus; nux vomica; phosphoricum acidum. Homeopathic hormones (e.g. testosterone, DHEA) may be prescribed by a qualified practitioner.

If at the end of the programme, there is no significant improvement in your sex drive, consult your doctor in case you need further investigations (e.g. prolactin or other hormone measurements) and treatment.

5. Over 45's prostate plan

Basic supplements to take throughout the programme:

- Multivitamin and mineral supplement designed for your age group.
- Evening primrose oil (1000mg per day) to provide the essential fatty acids, needed for synthesis and balance of sex hormones.
- Saw palmetto e.g. Formula 600 Plus for Men (FSC); Sabalin (Lichtwer Pharma/Medic Herb); Efaprost (Efamol); saw palmetto fruit extracts: 150mg – 3g daily in divided doses; products standardized for 85% – 95% fat-soluble sterols: 320mg daily.

Weeks 1 – 6: Touchfire His drops for men: 30 – 40 drops in water, twice daily (muira puama, catuaba, damiana, sarsaparilla, nettle root).

Weeks 7 – 12: If you have started to notice a benefit, continue with the supplements you are taking.

If you have not noticed a benefit, add in, or switch to, one or more of the following supplements having first read about them in the relevant chapter to see which would suit you best:

- Libido (chicken egg extracts): 6 capsules morning and evening for one week, then 2 capsules morning and evening thereafter
- L-arginine 150mg to 3g daily, ideally one hour before sex
- Korean ginseng: 600mg daily
- tribulus terrestris: 250mg
- ashwagandha: 150 – 300 mg
- bee pollen 250mg – 2g daily
- fo-ti 5g daily
- rye pollen extracts: one to two 252mg tablets daily for 6 weeks, after which you can reduce to one tablet per day for as long as required
- Love Life: 3 tablets twice a day
- Male Plus: 30 – 40 drops in water, twice a day

If you wish to use a homeopathic remedy, select one of the following, having first read Chapter 10: arsenicum album, conium maculatum; ferrum picricum; Love Life; lycopodium; populace tremuloides; homeopathic hormones (e.g. testosterone, DHEA) may be prescribed by a qualified practitioner.

NB men with prostate symptoms should continue to have a regular medical review of their condition.

If at the end of the programme, there is no significant improvement in your sex drive, consult your doctor in case you need further investigations (e.g. prolactin or other hormone measurements) and treatment.

6. Over 45's erectile dysfunction plan

Basic supplements to take throughout the programme:

- Multivitamin and mineral supplement designed for your age group.
- Evening primrose oil (1000mg per day) to provide the essential fatty acids, needed for synthesis and balance of sex hormones.
- Ginkgo biloba: Extracts standardized for at least 24% ginkolides: 40 – 60mg 2 to 3 times a day (take a minimum of 120mg daily).
- Consider taking Omega–3 fish oils and garlic powder tablets (e.g. Kwai One-a-day) to help maintain a healthy circulation including that to the penis.
- Consider taking Co-enzyme Q10 if lacking in energy.

Weeks 1 – 6: catuaba: 1g twice a day.

Weeks 7 – 12: If you have started to notice a benefit, continue with the supplements you are taking.

If you have not noticed a benefit, add in, or switch to, one or more of the following supplements having first read about them in the relevant chapter to see which would suit you best:

- Touchfire His drops for men: (Muira puama, catuaba, damiana, sarsaparilla and nettle root) 30 to 40 drops in water, twice a day
- Muira puama 1 – 1.5g daily for two weeks
- Libido (chicken egg extracts): 6 capsules morning and evening for one week, then 2 capsules morning and evening thereafter
- Korean ginseng 600mg daily for 6 weeks
- L-arginine 150mg to 3g daily, ideally one hour before sex
- DHEA or wild yam complexes designed to enhance natural DHEA production

- tribulus terrestris: 250mg daily
- fo-ti 5g daily
- ginger: 250mg two to four times
- sarsaparilla: 250mg three times a day
- ashwagandha: 150 – 300 mg
- bee pollen: 250mg – 2g daily
- Love Life: 3 tablets twice a day
- Male Plus: 30 – 40 drops in water, twice a day

If you wish to use a homeopathic remedy, select one of the following, having first read Chapter 10: Amphosca for Men; arsenicum album, baryta carbonica; conium maculatum; graphites; Love Life; lycopodium; plumbum metallicum; sulphur; homeopathic hormones (e.g. testosterone, DHEA) may be prescribed by a qualified practitioner.

If at the end of the programme, there is no significant improvement in your sex drive, consult your doctor in case you need further investigations (e.g. prolactin or other hormone measurements) and treatment.

WOMEN: Boost your sex drive

- Follow the diet and lifestyle plan at the beginning of this chapter, ensuring you have a good intake of vitamins and minerals.
- Use a vaginal lubricant (e.g. KY, Senselle, Replens or Sylk) – this is especially important during and after the menopause, if you are on the oral contraceptive Pill and after having a baby as vaginal lubrication is suppressed during breastfeeding.
- Consider using a pheromone preparation (see Chapter 5).
- If you wish to try aromatherapy, select essential oils from the charts and blends given in Chapter 11. If you are also

taking homeopathic remedies, do not use peppermint, rosemary or lavender essential oils as these may neutralize the homeopathic effect.

Follow one of six tailored programmes below, designed to suit the needs of:

1. Younger women with a low sex drive
2. Women whose low sex drive is linked with premenstrual syndrome
3. Women who have had a baby and are breastfeeding
4. Women who have had a baby but are not breastfeeding
5. Mature women during and after the menopause
6. Non-oestrogenic plan for women advised to avoid oestrogenic supplements (e.g. because of a potentially oestrogen-sensitive condition such as breast cancer).

Some supplements are available in health food stores or chemists, others by mail order (*see Resources*).

NB do not take herbal supplements if you are pregnant or planning to be, except under medical advice.

1. Young women's plan

Basic Supplements to take throughout the programme:

- A multivitamin and mineral supplement providing around 100% of the recommended daily amount (RDA) of as many micronutrients as possible, plus important trace elements such as boron, chromium, copper and molybdenum (e.g. Centrum). Blue-green algae is a suitable alternative if you prefer.
- Evening primrose oil (1000mg per day) to provide the essential fatty acids, needed for synthesis and balance of sex hormones.

- Siberian ginseng (eleutherococcus) capsules: 1g twice a day.
- Consider taking Co-enzyme Q10 if you feel lacking in energy.

Weeks 1 – 6: Touchfire Hers drops for women (chuchuhuasi, catuaba, damiana, suma, maca, sarsaparilla, abuta): 30 drops in water or juice, twice a day.

Weeks 7 – 12: If you have started to notice a benefit, continue with the supplements you are taking.

If you have not noticed a benefit, add in, or change to, one or more of the following supplements having first read about them in the relevant chapter to see which would suit you best:

- ashwagandha: 150 – 300mg daily
- Brazilian ginseng (pfaffia or suma): 1g daily
- catuaba: 1g twice a day
- gotu kola: 60 – 120mg daily
- guarana: 1g daily
- reishi: 500mg two to three times daily
- schisandra: 250mg – 500mg once to three times daily
- St.John's Wort: 300 – 600mg hypericins daily
- Intra (Healthcare International): 30ml daily
- oats (oatstraw): 3ml tincture, three times a day
- chicken egg extracts (Libido in UK, Ardor in US): 6 capsules twice daily for one week, then 1 capsule twice daily thereafter)
- fo-ti: 5g daily
- L-arginine: 150mg to 3g daily
- bee pollen: 250mg – 2g daily
- Love Life: 3 tablets twice a day
- Jaguara: 30 drops in water, twice a day

If you wish to use a homeopathic remedy, select one of the following, having first read Chapter 10: Amphosca for Women; arsenicum album; cactus grandiflorus; calcarea carbonica; cimicifuga; cuprum metallicum; folliculinum; gelsemium sempervirens; graphites; kali carbonicum; lachesis; lycopodium; natrum muriaticum; nux vomica; phosphoricum acidum; platinum metallicum; plumbum metallicum; pulsatilla nigricans; rhus toxicodenron; sepia; staphysagria; sulphur.

Homeopathic hormones (oestrogen, progesterone, testosterone; DHEA, thyroxine) are also available from practitioners (e.g. Wimbledon Clinic of Natural Medicine – *see Resources*).

If at the end of the programme there is no significant improvement in your sex drive, consult your doctor in case you need further investigations (e.g. prolactin or other hormone measurements) and treatment.

2. Premenstrual syndrome plan

Basic Supplements to take throughout the programme:

- A multivitamin and mineral supplement providing around 100% of the recommended daily amount (RDA) of as many micronutrients as possible, plus important trace elements such as boron, chromium, copper and molybdenum (e.g. Centrum). Blue-green algae is a suitable alternative if you prefer.
- Evening primrose oil (3g per day) to provide the essential fatty acids needed for synthesis and balance of sex hormones.

Weeks 1 – 6: agnus castus: 500mg daily
Weeks 7 – 12: If you have started to notice a benefit, continue with the supplements you are taking.

If you have not noticed a benefit, add in, or change to, one or more of the following supplements having first read about them in the relevant chapter to see which would suit you best:

- Touchfire Hers drops for women (chuchuhuasi, catuaba, damiana, suma, maca, sarsaparilla, abuta): 30 drops in water or juice, twice a day
- black cohosh: 2ml tincture, twice daily
- chicken egg extracts (Libido in UK, Ardor in US): 6 capsules twice daily for one week, then 1 capsule twice daily thereafter)
- dong quai: 500mg daily
- red clover: 500mg daily
- Siberian ginseng
- wild Yam: 250 – 500 mg
- muira puama 1 – 1.5g daily for two weeks
- bee pollen: 250mg – 2g daily
- Love Life: 3 tablets twice a day
- Jaguara: 30 drops in water, twice a day

If you wish to use a homeopathic remedy, select one of the following, having first read Chapter 10: Amphosca for Women; arsenicum album; Bach Rescue Remedy; cactus grandiflorus; calcarea carbonica; cimicifuga; folliculinum; lachesis; Love Life; platinum metallicum; pulsatilla nigricans; rhus toxicodendron; sepia. Homeopathic hormones (oestrogen, progesterone, testosterone; DHEA, thyroxine) are also available from practitioners (e.g. Wimbledon Clinic of Natural Medicine see *Resources*).

You may also wish to consider using progesterone cream (*see page 106*).

If at the end of the programme, there is no significant improvement in your sex drive, consult your doctor in case you need further investigations (e.g. prolactin or other hormone measurements) and treatment, having first read about them in the relevant chapter to see which would suit you best:

Postnatal plan

Read information on prolactin hormone and the reasons for low sex drive after childbirth, especially when breastfeeding. It helps to know that postnatal loss of sex drive is normal and predictable. Hormone changes will not affect your ability to achieve and enjoy an orgasm, however, so try to get in the right mood for making love by using sensual aromatherapy oils to scent your bedroom. Do not massage essential oils onto your skin if you are breastfeeding except under the advice of a qualified aromatherapist.

Massage the area between the vagina and back passage (perineum) with an antenatal massage cream or oil daily.

3. Breastfeeding plan

Basic Supplements to take throughout the programme:

- Multivitamin and mineral supplement designed for pregnancy and breastfeeding (e.g. ProNatal).
- Essential fatty acid supplement designed for pregnancy and breastfeeding (e.g. EfaNatal or Milkarra in the UK; Neuromins in the US) OR evening primrose oil 3g daily.
- Consider taking Co-enzyme Q10 if you feel lacking in energy.

Weeks 1 – 6: agnus castus: 500mg daily (stimulates milk production and boosts libido – but do not take if using the mini-Pill – take oats instead, in this case).

Weeks 7 – 12: If you have started to notice a benefit, continue with the supplements you are taking.

If you have not noticed a benefit, add in one or more of the following supplements having first read about them in the relevant chapter to see which would suit you best:

- oats (oatstraw): 1 dropperful fluid-extract or tincture two or three times daily.
- abuta (check dose).
- cayenne: 2ml tincture.
- garlic: Kwai One-a-Day.
- ginger: 250mg four times daily.

4. NOT breastfeeding

Basic Supplements to take throughout the programme:

- Multivitamin and mineral supplement designed for pregnancy and afterwards (e.g. ProNatal).
- evening primrose oil 3g daily.
- Consider taking Co-enzyme Q10 if you feel lacking in energy.

Weeks 1 – 6: St. John's Wort: Extracts standardized for hypericin: 300 – 600 micrograms hypericin three times daily. (lowers prolactin levels, so only use if not breastfeeding)

Weeks 7 – 12: If you have started to notice a benefit, continue with the supplements you are taking.

If you have not noticed a benefit, add in one or more of the following supplements having first read about them in the relevant chapter to see which would suit you best:

- sage (reduces milk flow during weaning): Tincture 3ml with water twice a day
- Touchfire Hers drops for women (chuchuhuasi catuaba, damiana, suma, maca, sarsaparilla, abuta)
- chicken egg extracts (6 capsules twice a day for morning and evening for one week, then 2 capsules morning and evening thereafter)
- Brazilian ginseng (pfaffia or suma): 1g daily

- Siberian ginseng (eleutherococcus) capsules: 1g twice a day
- Intra (Healthcare International) 30ml daily
- bee pollen: 250mg – 2g daily
- Long life: 3 tablets twice a day
- Jaguara: 30 drops in water, twice a day

If low sex drive is linked with postnatal depression, you must seek medical help from your doctor, midwife or health visitor immediately.

If you wish to use a homeopathic remedy as part of your postnatal programme, select one of the following, having first read Chapter 10: cimicifuga; graphites; kali carbonicum; Love Life; lycopodium; natrum muriaticum; phosphoricum acidum; platinum metallicum; plumbum metallicum; rhus toxicodenron; sepia; staphysagria (especially if you have had a Caesarean). If you are breastfeeding, consult a homeopath first.

If at the end of the programme, there is no significant improvement in your sex drive, try not to worry unduly. Sex drive can take a while to return to normal, as prolactin levels slowly fall (*see page 22*) especially if breastfeeding. Persevere with the programme for a little longer as your sex drive will slowly start to return. If, after trying a number of remedies, you are still unhappy – don't be afraid to consult your doctor.

5. Menopausal plan

Basic Supplements to take throughout the programme:

- A multivitamin and mineral supplement specifically designed for your age group that includes important trace elements such as boron, chromium, copper and molybdenum. Blue-green algae is a suitable alternative if you prefer.
- evening primrose oil (1g to 3g) daily.
- red clover: 500mg tablet or soy extracts (providing at least 50mg isoflavones a day).

- consider taking Co-enzyme Q10 if you feel lacking in energy.

Weeks 1 – 6: pfaffia (Brazilian ginseng or suma): 1g a day.
Weeks 7 – 12: If you have started to notice a benefit, continue with the supplements you are taking

If you have not noticed a benefit, add in one or more of the following supplements having first read about them in the relevant chapter to see which would suit you best:

- Siberian ginseng: 1 to 2g daily
- dong quai: 500mg daily
- black cohosh: Tincture: 2–4ml daily
- St. John's Wort: Extracts standardized for hypericin: 300 – 600 micrograms hypericin three times daily
- wild Yam: 250 – 500 mg
- ginkgo biloba: take a minimum of 120mg daily
- kava kava: 100mg three times daily
- agnus castus: 500mg daily
- chicken egg extracts: 6 capsules twice a day for one week then 1 capsule twice a day thereafter
- damiana: 400mg daily
- gotu kola: 60 – 120mg daily
- false unicorn root: 10 drops tincture, three times a day
- Royal jelly: 50 to 100mg per day
- bee pollen: 250mg – 2g daily
- sage: Tincture: 4ml daily
- Long life: 3 tablets twice a day
- Jaguara: 30 drops in water, twice a day

Consider using a progesterone cream.

If you wish to use a homeopathic remedy, select one of the following, having first read Chapter 10: agnus castus; Amphosca for

Women; cactus grandiflorus; calcarea carbonica; cimicifuga; gelsemium sempervirens; graphites; kali carbonicum; lachesis; Love Life; lycopodium; natrum muriaticum; nux vomica; phosphoricum acidum; platinum metallicum; plumbum metallicum; pulsatilla nigricans; rhus toxicodenron; sepia; staphysagria (especially if you have had a hysterectomy) sulphur.

Homeopathic hormones (oestrogen, progesterone, testosterone; DHEA, thyroxine) are also available from practitioners (e.g. Wimbledon Clinic of Natural Medicine see Resources).

If at the end of the programme, there is no significant improvement in your sex drive, consult your doctor in case you need further investigations or treatment.

You may wish to consider taking hormone replacement therapy (HRT). In some cases, treatment with DHEA, testosterone or tibolone may be suggested (*see Chapter 8*).

6. Non-oestrogenic plan

Basic Supplements to take throughout the programme:

- a multivitamin and mineral supplement specifically designed for your age group that includes important trace elements such as boron, chromium, copper and molybdenum. Blue-green algae is a suitable alternative if you prefer
- evening primrose oil (1g) daily
- Consider taking milk thistle to improve liver function: 200mg three times daily.

Weeks 1 – 6: agnus castus: 500mg daily
Weeks 7 – 12: If you have started to notice a benefit, continue with the supplements you are taking.

If you have not noticed a benefit, add in one or more of the following supplements having first read about them in the relevant chapter to see which would suit you best:

- St.John's Wort: Extracts standardized for hypericin: 300 – 600 micrograms hypericin three times daily
- reishi: 500mg three times daily
- black cohosh: standardized to provide 27-deoxyacteine: 1-2mg twice daily (or tincture 4ml daily (because its unique action does not stimulate oestrogen-sensitive tumours, and may even inhibit them, black cohosh has been used in women with a history of breast cancer)
- sarsaparilla: 250mg three times daily
- ginkgo: at least 120mg daily
- catuaba: 1gm twice a day
- damiana: 400mg daily
- fo-ti: 5g daily
- wild yam: 500mg daily

If you wish to use a homeopathic remedy, select one of the following, having first read Chapter 10: agnus castus; Amphosca for Women; cimicifuga; graphites; kali carbonicum; lachesis; Love Life; lycopodium; natrum muriaticum; phosphoricum acidum; platinum metallicum; plumbum metallicum; pulsatilla nigricans; rhus toxicodenron; sepia; staphysagria (especially if you have had surgery); sulphur.

Homeopathic hormones (progesterone, testosterone; DHEA, thyroxine) are also available from practitioners (e.g. Wimbledon Clinic of Natural Medicine *see Resources*).

If at the end of the programme there is no significant improvement in your sex drive, consult your doctor in case you need further investigations or treatment. In some cases, treatment with progesterone, DHEA, testosterone or tibolone may be suggested (*see Chapter 8*).

Case Histories

Scott, 33, is happily married with two children. He enjoys his work as a salesman and does not feel particularly stressed. Six months ago, he developed a low sex drive that came on suddenly – he just lost interest in sex. It wasn't a problem for him, but his wife Lindsay began to wonder if he was having an affair at work. At first Scott refused to seek help – partly because it was an embarrassing topic to discuss with his GP, and partly because having a low sex drive did not particularly bother him. Eventually he agreed to seek help when he realised his marriage was at risk. At first, his doctor advised him to stop drinking, take a vitamin and mineral supplement, and to increase his level of exercise. When Scott developed low grade headaches, his GP performed a blood test to measure levels of prolactin hormone. They were sky high. A skull X-ray and subsequent brain scan confirmed that Scott had a prolactinoma – a benign tumour of the pituitary gland. Scott was seen by a neurosurgeon who initially prescribed bromocriptine tablets. This brought the prolactin levels down to almost the normal range. Scott is now under regular review – if the tumour grows any larger, he will need surgery to remove the tumour. Although his sex drive has now improved, the worry about his condition means it has still not returned to its previous levels.

Ricardo, 29, has a high powered financial job in the City. He works long hours, is under stress, drinks excessive amounts of alcohol and smokes heavily. He freely admits his lifestyle is a mess. He kept meaning to do something about it, but was always too busy. He usually had at least one girlfriend in tow, but relationships did not usually last long because he slowly became less and less interested in sex. When he realised he had gone for six weeks without sex – yet was not champing at the bit as he would have expected – he realised something was wrong. Ricardo started a programme involving a vitamin and mineral supplement, reducing his intake of alcohol and trying to stop smoking. Having read about pro-sexual supplements he decided to take tincture of oats (which also helped to reduce his nicotine cravings), Libido (chicken egg extracts) and decided to add in Korean ginseng as well, mainly because a friend was taking it and noticed increased energy reserves. Within two weeks, Ricardo started to experience sexual urges again, and was back to normal within a month.

John, 49, has diabetes and found that it was increasingly difficult to maintain an erection. His desire for sex had also decreased and this was putting a strain on his marriage. He started to take ginkgo biloba, garlic powder tablets and fish oil supplements to improve his circulation, and after a month noticed a significant improvement in erectile rigidity. His libido was still low however, so he added in catuaba. He was amazed at the effect and he claims his sex life is now better than in his youth.

David, 57, has developed symptoms of prostatism that wake him at night to pass water. His ability to maintain an erection has also decreased and his desire for sex reduced – mostly because of fear of failure. His wife bought him some saw palmetto, having read about it in a magazine. After taking it for six weeks, his prostate symptoms were significantly improved. He and his wife then both started taking Touchfire His and Hers drops and have noticed a definite improvement in both their sex drives.

Paul, 30, is in a relationship with an Italian woman who has an unusually high sex drive. At first, he found this exciting, but started to feel pressurized into having sex when he wasn't ready. A friend suggested that he tried muira puama – and jokingly referred to it as nature's Viagra. He took one course for ten days and noticed an instant reaction. He did not need to take it again for three months.

Jason, 25, is gay and in a stable relationship. He works long hours and has found that, after the initial excitement of falling in love, his desire for sex has diminished. Both he and his partner started to take Viryl-forte plus L-arginine and have noticed a marked increase in sexual desire.

Becky, 29, has two small children and often goes to bed feeling too exhausted for sex. Her husband has a relatively high sex drive, and Becky was starting to resent his continued demands for sex. Realizing that they were developing a serious problem, she started to take a vitamin and mineral supplement, plus co-enzyme Q10 for extra energy. She then started taking Jaguara Amazon Formula for Women and added in evening primrose oil. After six weeks, she felt more interested in sex and no longer resented her husband's advances. On the suggestion of her doctor, she then started taking St John's Wort as well as he felt she was mildly depressed. Becky no longer feels exhausted when going to bed, and recently surprised both herself and her husband by initiating sex herself rather than waiting for him to make the first move.

Sara, 32, has premenstrual syndrome and for half of each month, has no interest in sex. She has a long-suffering boyfriend who is supportive but she realizes that their relationship is under strain because of her recurrent monthly symptoms. She takes vitamin B_6, evening primrose oil and a magnesium supplement but although these help her physical symptoms, have not improved her sex drive. Sara started to take agnus castus regularly, and also Amphosca for women. Although she still has several days just before each period when she feels too bloated to enjoy sex, her libido has returned.

Lucy, 26, has just had her first baby. She has been breastfeeding for four months and hopes to continue until baby Anna is at least a year old. Lucy's sex drive has still not returned, and her midwife explained this was due to the effects of prolactin hormone. She is still taking ProNatal vitamin and mineral supplement, plus Efanatal for essential fatty acids. On the advice of her midwife, she added in agnus castus and has found that not only has her milk production increased, but her sex drive is returning as well.

Pritha, 27, has also just had a baby and found her sex drive is non-existent. This has been made worse by the fact that she could not breastfeed properly as the baby continually failed to latch on. Following a breast abscess resulting from milk engorgement, Pritha developed postnatal depression. Her herbalist advised taking St John's Wort to lift her mood, and sage to reduce milk secretion. After two weeks, she stopped the sage as her breasts were feeling more comfortable, and started taking Siberian ginseng. Her sex drive started to return within two weeks and is now back to normal.

Jennifer, 53, found her sex drive disappeared when her periods stopped a year previously. At first this wasn't a problem as she wasn't in a relationship. Once she met a potential partner however, she realised she would have to do something about it. Her doctor pre-scribed hormone replacement therapy and her libido came back quite strongly. She developed migraine however and the HRT was stopped, at which point her sex drive dwindled again. She started taking red clover extracts and noticed that both her hot flushes reduced and her libido returned within two weeks.

Simone, 49, also developed low sex drive at the menopause, but was unwilling to take hormone replacement therapy due to a strong family history of breast cancer. She was advised to take black cohosh and also used a wild yam cream. Within a month, her menopausal symptoms had improved and her sex drive was picking up. She added a Pheromone product to her favourite perfume, Opium, and noticed that male friends were more attentive which in turn made her feel more attractive and sexy herself.

Anne and Nick, both in their 40's, decided to go on a second honeymoon once their children had left home. Their sex life had become jaded and they only indulged once or twice a month. They read about the combined tablet and homeopathic tincture programme, Love Life, and decided to start taking it before they went away. As well as pepping up their sex drive, they found the fun of taking the tablets and comparing notes on the effects brought them closer together. Both agreed it gave their libido a significant boost.

Resources

The Nutri Centre
The Hale Clinic
7 Park Crescent
London WIN 3HE
Tel: 0171 436 5122
Supply: Many of the general, herbal and homeopathic supplements mentioned in this book by mail order.

Supplements

Arkopharma
6 Redlands Centre
Redlands
Coulsdon
Surrey CR5 2HT
Tel: 0181 763 1414; fax: 0181 736 2124
Supply: Phytoforce: Siberian ginseng

Bioforce UK Ltd
2 Brewster Place
Irvine
Ayrshire KA11 5DD
Tel: 01294 277344; fax: 01294 277922
Supply: Agnus castus, Avena sativa (oat seed), eleutherococcus (Siberian ginseng), Ginkgo biloba, hypericum perforatum, menosan (sage), urtica dioica (stinging nettle), valeriana, melissa officinalis (lemon balm), milk thistle complex, saw palmetto complex, Jan de Vries Emergency Essence, ginger, kava kava.

Blackmores
Tel: 0181 987 8640; fax: 0181 987 8641
Supply: 45 Plus: menopausal supplement containing dong quai and black cohosh; Phytolife Plus: soy extracts containing isoflavones; Active Woman Formula: includes Siberian ginseng, wild oats, damiana and gotu kola.

Bodyonics
140 Lauman Lane
Hicksville
New York 11801
Tel: 1 800 527 7965; Outside US: 1 516 822 1230
Supply: Tribestrol: tribulus terrestris

Britannia Health Products Ltd
41–51 Brighton Road
Redhill
Surrey RH1 6YS
Tel: 01737 773741; fax: 01737 762672
Supply: ProstaBrit: rye pollen extracts

English Grains Healthcare
William Nadin Way
Swadlincote
Derbyshire DE11 0BB
Produce: Red Kooga ginseng.

Efamol Ltd
Weyvern House
Weyvern Park
Portsmouth Road
Peasmarsh
Guildford
Surrey GU3 1NA
Tel: 01483 304441; fax: 01483 304437; order line: 0800 318545.
Supply: Efamol evening primrose oil; Efanatal (evening primrose oil plus fish oils) for women who are pregnant or breastfeeding; Efaprost: containing evening primrose oil, saw palmetto, beta-sitosterol for men.

Enzymatic Therapy
Green Bay
Wisconsin 54311
Tel: 1 414 469 1313
Supply: Remifemin (a standardized extract of black cohosh).

Futurebiotics
Hauppauge
New York
Tel: 1–800-FOR LIFE; Internet: www.futurebiotics.com.
Supply: Male Power, a male energising formula: contains Korean ginseng, wild oats, saw palmetto, fo-ti, schisandra, deer antler, bee pollen, Siberian ginseng, wild yam, astragalus, black cohosh, ginger,

royal jelly and glandular extracts; Maxativa, a sensual herb formula for men: contains wild oats, sarsaparilla, ginseng, damiana, nettles, bee pollen, royal jelly, zinc and B_3; Maxativa for Women, a sensual herb formula for women: contains vitamins, minerals, suma, wild yam, Korean ginseng, choline, damiana, ginger, wild oats.

Health & Diet Company
Europa Park
Radcliffe
Manchester M26 1GG
Tel: 01204 707420; fax: 01204 792238
Supply: FSC Herbcraft ranges (tinctures & capsules); Formula 600 Plus for men: contains zinc, Vitamin B_6, copper, saw palmetto, pygeum africanum and pumpkin powder, cayenne and amino acids; agnus castus premenstrual tincture; black cohosh and wild yam menopause tincture; ginkgo biloba plus tincture; ginseng & saw palmetto for men tincture; reishi shiitake mushrooms tincture; saw palmetto plus tincture and tablets; agnus castus tincture & tablets; cayenne tincture; dong quai tincture; garlic tincture; ginkgo biloba tincture; gotu kola tincture & tablets; kava kava tincture & tablets; milk thistle tincture & tablets; Siberian ginseng tincture & tablets; St John's Wort tincture & tablets; wild yam tincture; black cohosh; dong quai; damiana; fo-ti tieng; ginkgo biloba; ginger; ginger & turmeric; Korean ginseng; nettles; passionflower; sarsaparilla; wild yam; fresh royal jelly; Co-enzyme Q10.

Healthcare International
18 St Peter's Avenue
Witherley
Leicestershire CV9 3LN
Tel: 01827 716918

Supply: Intra: a liquid supplement containing a variety of adaptogenic and pro-sexual herbs including schisandra, reishi, bee pollen, passion flower, ginger, sarsaparilla, astragalus and Siberian ginseng in a base of grape/pear juice.

Kordel Healthcare Ltd
Bradford Yorks
Tel: 01274 488511

Kordel (Australia) PTY Ltd
102 Bath Road
Kirrawee, NSW

Health Foods International Ltd
9 Canon Place
Pakuranga
Auckland
Supply: Zest for Men: contains zinc and other vitamins, minerals and trace elements; damiana, Siberian ginseng, oyster extract, sarsaparilla, saw palmetto, cayenne.

Health of the Nation
Kingfisher
Swancraft Marina
Henley Rad
Wargrave
Berks RG10 8HZ
Tel/fax: 0118 940 1794
Supply: Love Life tablets: contains the oriental herbs rehmannia, astragalus, dong quai, atractyloides, lycii, polygonum, merinda, cistanches, epimedium, allium, curculigo, dioscorea, cuscutea, achyranthes, paeonia alba, polygola, Korean ginseng, cnidium, poria cocos,

cinnamon, eucomia cornus plus vitamins A, B_1, B_2, B_3, B_5, B_6, B_{12}, folic acid, and minerals boron, copper, magnesium, selenium and zinc; Love Life Homeopathic tincture: contains agnus castus, American arum, baryta carb, cinchone, sepia, selenium, phosphorica.

Herbal Alternative Laboratories Ltd
Lime Tree House
Lime Tree Walk
Sevenoaks
Kent TN13 1YH
Tel: 07132 746604; fax: 01732 465500. Order number at JEM Marketing: 01483 204417; e-mail: herballabs@hotmail.com
Supply: Herbal V: contains Muira puama.

Immuno Vital Inc.
PO Box 450097
Miami
Florida 33245
USA
Supply: Maca

Larkhall Green Farm
225 Putney Bridge Road
London SW15 2PY
Tel: 0181 874 1130; fax: 0181 871 0066
Supply: Cantassium, Nature's Plus and Natural Flow ranges; Viryl-Forte: contains L-arginine, L-histidine, zinc, Korean ginseng, damiana, niacin; L-arginine; L-histidine; L-tyrosine; DL-phenylalanine; royal jelly; Co-enzyme Q10; agnus castus; ginger herbal; ginkgo biloba; ginseng red panax; propolis; royal jelly; tong kwai (dong quai); triple ginseng; Liv-R-Actin (milk thistle containing silymarin);

suma; Sylk personal lubricant; Rise Cream for Men; Vaccuum Developer 6–8; Bliss Cream for Women.

Lichtwer Pharma UK Ltd/Medic Herb
Regency House
Mere Park
Dedmere Road
Marlow
Bucks SL7 1FJ
Tel: 01628 487780; fax: 01628 487781
Supply: Sabalin – standardized saw palmetto; Ginkyo – standardized ginkgo; Kwai – standardized, powdered garlic tablets; kira – standardized St John's wort; Valerina Daytime and Valerina Night-time (Valarian and Melissa relaxing herbs).

Life Enhancement Products Inc.
1340 Industrial Ave
Suite A
Petaluma, CA 94952
Toll Free: 1 800 543 3873; outside US Tel: 1 707 762 6144; Fax: 1 769 8016; Internet: www.life-enhancement.com
Supply: ProSexual Plus: vitamins, minerals, arginine and ginkgo, yohimbe tonic, saw palmetto.

Life Plus Europe Ltd
Martin House
Howard Road
Eaton Socon
Cambs PE19 3ET
Tel: 01480 477230; Fax: 01480 403772

Life Plus USA
Box 3749
Batesville
AR 72503, USA
Tel 800 572 8446
Supply: Touchfire His Drops for Men – liquid herbal extracts of Muira puama (potency wood), catuaba, damiana, sarsaparilla and nettle root); Touchfire Hers drops for Women – liquid herbal extracts of chuchuhuasi, catuaba, damiana, suma, maca, sarsaparilla, abuta; Co-enzyme Q10 Plus; Prostate Formula: contains saw palmetto, jatoba and pau d'arco.

Nature's Remedies Ltd
15 Little End Road
Eaton Socon
Cambridgeshire
PE19 3JH
Tel: 01480 403768; fax: 01480 403757
Supply: Male Plus Amazon herbal formula for men: contains Muira puama, catuaba, damiana, sarsaparilla; Jaguara for women: contains chuchuhuas, catuaba, maca, abuta, damiana. Also supply a variety of other herbs from the rainforest.

Novogen Ltd
140 Wicks Road
North Ryde
NSW 2113
Australia
Tel: 61 2 9878 0088 Fax: 61 2 9878 0055
Supply: Promensil: red clover extracts

Novus Research
Tel: 888–872–8893
Supply: PRO-Symbio HGH: growth hormone releaser (arginine, glutamine, ornithine and lysine).

PharmaNord (UK) Ltd
Spital Hall
Mitford Morpeth
NE61 3PN
Tel: 01670 519989 Fax: 01670 513222
Supply: Bio-Quinone Q10; bio-biloba.

Quest Vitamins Ltd
8 Venture Way
Aston Science Park
Birmingham, B7 4AP
Tel: 0121 359 0056; Fax: 0121–359 0313; e-mail: info@questvitamins.co.uk
Supply: Agnus castus; St John's Wort; Siberian ginseng; saw palmetto; milk thistle; ginger; L-arginine; L-phenylalanine; L-tyrosine.

Raintree Group
2949 West Anderson Lane
Suite 175
Austin Texas 78757
Tel: 512 467 6130
Supply: Male Plus: herbal supplement including damiana and sarsaparilla, suma.

Rio Trading
2 Centenary Estate
Brighton
East Sussex BN2 4AW
Tel: 01273 570987
Supply: Love Gum: contains Siberian ginseng; catuaba; Brazilian ginseng (Pfaffia); guarana.

Solgar Vitamins Ltd
Aldbury
Tring
Herts HP23 5PT
Tel: 01442 890355; fax: 01442 890366
Supply: Gold Label Range: American ginseng; black cohosh; cayenne; dong quai; ginkgo biloba; gotu kola; kava kava; Korean ginseng; milk thistle; red clover leaf extract; sarsaparilla; saw palmetto; Siberian ginseng; St John's wort; L-arginine; histidine Complex tablets; L-phenylalanine; L-tyrosine; Phosphatidyl-choline; Co-Enzyme Q10; bee pollen; reishi shiitake maitake extracts.

Tree of Life
1750 Tree Boulevard
St Augustines
Florida 32087 Tel: 904–824–8181
and
NewYouth
Balara Bay
Governor's Harbour
Eleuthera, Bahamas
Tel: 001–242–332–2700; Fax: 001–242–332–2388; e-mail: newyouth@batelnet.bs
and

Medical Innovations
Newlands Medical Centres
315 Chorley New Road
Bolton BL1 5BP
Tel: 01204 842830; fax: 01204 847073
Supply: Ardor (US) chicken egg extracts; Libido (UK) chicken egg extracts.

Xynergy Health Products
Lower Elsted
Midhurst
West Sussex GU29 0JT.
Tel: 01730 813642; Freephone: 0800 3760042; fax: 01730 815109

HC 64
Box 2901 Castle Valley
Utah 84532–9613
Supply: Pure Synergy: a blend of more than 60 energy-yielding superfoods (many of which are prosexual) including blue-green algae, Siberian ginseng, schisandra, ginger, astragalus, green juices, gingko, reishi, shiitake, papaya, royal jelly and natural antioxidants. Take one tablespoon of powder daily in a glass of water or fresh juice.

Hormone Stimulating Supplements

DHEA and related products may be imported into the UK by mail order for personal use only. Packages may be opened by Customs, but will be resealed and forwarded. NB: DHEA is classed as a controlled drug in some countries such as Canada, so that its importation and possession is illegal.

Wild yam products that contain substances which may boost hormone production are available in the UK. While they may not be as effective as hormonal preparations, they have the advantage of few side effects.

Futurebiotics
Hauppauge
New York
Tel: 1 800-FOR-LIFE; Internet: www.futurebiotics.com
Supply: DHEA: hormonal DHEA

Life Enhancement Products Inc.
1340 Industrial Ave
Suite A
Petaluma
CA 94952
Toll Free: 1 800 543 3873; Outside US Tel: 1 707 762 6144; Fax: 1 769 8016; Internet: www.life-enhancement.com
Supply: DHEA test kits; DHEA: hormonal DHEA; InnerPower: growth hormone releaser; pregnenolone; ginkgo; progesterone-transdermal; progesterone DP (with DHEA and Pregnenolone).

Books

Better Sex Through Chemistry, Morgenthaler & Joy (Smart Publications, California, USA)
Natural Hormone Replacement, Wright & Morgenthaler (Smart Publications, California, USA)
Smart Drugs & Nutrients, Dean & Morgenthaler (Smart Publications, California, USA)
Smart Drugs II, Dean, Morgenthaler & Fowkes (Smart Publications, California, USA)

Life Plus USA
Box 3749
Batesville
AR 72503, USA
Tel 800 572 8446
Supply: Endocryn DHEA: hormonal DHEA

Natural Balance
PO Box 8002
Castle Rock
CO 80104 8002, USA
Tel: 800 833 8737; 303 688 6633; Fax: 303 688 1591
Supply: DHEA Super Hormone: hormonal DHEA; DHEA Super Hormone for Men: DHEA plus zinc in a herbal base containing yohimbe, guarana, Korean ginseng; horny goat weed; Muira puama and catuaba; Andro-Max: androstenedione and tribulus terrestris; pregnenolone; pregnenolone with DHEA.

Nutrapharm
PO Box 12811
London N20 9WA
Tel: 0181 492 0044; Fax: 0181 446 5119
and
Neutraceutics Corporation, USA
Supply: Pro-Estron: conjugated phytoestrogenic complex; DHEA Plus/Vita DHEA: herbal wild yam complex designed to boost natural production of DHEA; Testron SX: herbal wild yam complex designed to boost natural production of testosterone, Pro-hGH: natural complexes designed to boost production of growth hormone; pure royal jelly; DH3: ginkgo, B_{12} and wild yam.

Humanetics corporation
600 South Highway 169
Suite 1205, Minneapolis
MN 55426, US
Tel: 1 888 436 3584
Supply: 7-Keto-DHEA; pheromones

Larkhall Green Farm
225 Putney Bridge Road
London SW15 2PY
Tel: 0181 874 1130

Athena Institute for Women's Wellness Inc.
Chester Springs
Pennsylvania
Tel: 610 827 2200 PA 19041
Supply: Athena Pheromone 10:13 for Women; Athena Pheromone 10X for Men.

Pacific Sensuals
1414 S. Beverly Glen Blvd
Los Angeles; CA 90024
Tel: 310 286 1183; fax: 310 286 1184
Supply: Amate bark paper handmade candles: pheromone candles; Allure: pheromone massage oil; Erotikava: drink containing kava and an Asian herbal sensual tonic.

Homeopathy

Nutri-Centre
7 Park Crescent
London W1N 3HE
Tel: 0171 436 5122
and
Enzymatic Therapy
Green Bay
Wisconsin 54311
Tel: 414 469 1313
Supply: Amphosca for men; Amphosca for women

Biomed Comm, Inc.
2 Nickerson Ts
Suite 102
Seattle, WA 98109 Tel: 1 888 637 3516; fax: 206 284 3433
Supply: Homeopathic growth hormone

Homeopathic hormones are prescribed on an individual basis at:
The Wimbledon Clinic of Natural Medicine
1 Evelyn Road
London SW19 8NU
Tel: 0181 540 3389

Aromatherapy

Body Treats
Tel 0181 543 7633
Natural by Nature Oils
Tel 0181 202 5718

HelpLines

Efamol (Evening primrose oil) information line: 01483 570248

Garlic Information Centre: 01424 892440

Gingko Information Centre: 01424 892440

National alcohol helpline: 0345 320202

Drinkline: 0171–332 0202 (London only); 0345 320202 (nation-wide)
All calls charged at local rates.

Dial and listen: 0500 801802 FREECALL

Smokers' Quitline: 071 487 3000 (09.30 – 17.30 daily)

Logado (aromatherapy advice) Consumer Advice Line: 01223 426410

Men's Health Matters Adviceline: 0181 995 4448 (Mon-Fri 6pm – 10pm).

Freephone Cancer Information Helpline: 0800 132905

Miscellaneous

Aquaflex (vaginal cones that make pelvic floor exercises more effective): Freephone 0800 526177 to order or to speak to a trained nurse counsellor in confidence.

Sylk: a natural, vaginal lubrication derived from Kiwi fruit available by mail order only. SYLK Ltd, Freepost PO Box 340, Rickmansworth, Herts WD3 5WD. Tel: 01923 285544.

Counselling

British Association of Art Therapists
11a Richmond Road
Brighton
Sussex BN2 3RL

British Association for Behavioural Psychotherapy
Social Services Department
7 Whittaker Street
Radcliffe
Manchester M26 9TD

British Association for Counselling
1 Regent Place
Rugby Warwickshire CV21 2PJ
Tel: 01788 578328; send an SAE for a register of local accredited counsellors and a publication list.

British Association for Sexual and Marital Therapy
PO Box 13686
London SW20 9ZH
British Confederation of Psychotherapists
37 Mapesbury Road
London NW2 4HJ
Tel: 0181 830 5173
Provides a register of psychotherapists and a free brochure, *Finding a Therapist*.

British Psychological Society
St Andrew's House
48 Princess Road East
Leicester LE1 7DR
Tel: 0116 254 9568
Holds a register of Chartered Psychologists

Institute of Group Analysis
1 Daleham Gardens
London NW3 5BY
Tel: 0171–431–2693
Holds a list of qualified group analysts

British Association for the Person-Centred Approach
BM BAPCA
London WC1N 3XX

Institute for Transactional Analysis
BM Box 4104
London WC1N 3XX

Relate
Herbert Gray College
Little Church Street
Rugby
Warwickshire CV21 3AP
Tel: 01788–573241; fax: 01788–535007
Works to support marriage and family life by providing counselling
and sex therapy for couples with relationship problems, at over 120
local Centres nationwide.

Useful Organisations

Cancer BACUP
3 Bath Place
Rivington Street
London EC2A 3JR
Freeline: 0800 181199; Counselling: 0171 696 9000
Has produced a booklet, *Sexuality and Cancer*.

British Herbal Medicine Association
Sun House
Church St
Stroud GL5 1JL
Tel: 01453 751389
Information leaflets, booklets, compendium, telephone advice.

British Homeopathic Association
27A Devonshire Street
London W1N 1RJ
Tel: 0171 935 2163 (1.30 – 5.30 pm)
Leaflets, referral to medically qualified homeopathic doctors.

Depression Alliance
PO Box 1022
London SE1 7QB
Tel: 0171 721 7672 (answerphone only)
Has produced a leaflet *Depression & Your Sex life*.

General Council and Register of Naturopaths
Frazer House
6 Netherall Gardens
London NW3 5RR
0171–435–8728

International Stress Management Association
The Priory Hospital
Priory lane
London SW15 5JJ
Tel: 081 876 8261
Information on stress management and control. Leaflets, booklets, counselling.

Men's Health Matters
100 Blythe Road
London W14 0HB
Adviceline: 0181 995 4448 (Mon – Fri, 6pm – 10pm)
Provides information and advice on a range of male health problems, including prostate conditions and erectile dysfunction.

UK Sports Council,
Walkden House
10 Meldon Street
London NW1 2EB
Drug Information Line: 0171 380 8030.

SPOD (Sexual and Personal Relationships of People with a Disability)
286 Camden Road
London N7 0BJ
Tel: 0171 607 8851 (tues/thurs 10.30am – 1.30 pm; weds: 1.30pm – 4.30 pm).

Impotence Asociation
PO Box 10296
London SW17 9WH
Confidential Helpline: 0181–767–7791 9am – 5pm.
Please send a large stamped SAE for a leaflet: *Impotence explained – A Couples' Guide to Erectile Dysfunction*.

The Soil Association
40–56 Victoria Street,
Bristol
BS1 6BY
Tel: 0117 929 0661; Fax: 0117 925 2504
Produces a directory of local organic delivery services for a small fee.

Index

psychotherapy, 236–37
  person-centred, 237–38
  art, 238
pulsatilla nigricans, 184

recipes
  sexy weekend diet for two, 85–86
red clover, 155–56
reishi, 156–57
relaxation
  and health, 247
  techniques, 222–23
  activating the tan tien, 225
  mantra meditation, 224–5
  whole body, 223–4
  yoga breathing exercise, 224
rhus toxicodendron, 184–85
rose, 204
rosemary, 204–5
rosewood, 205
royal jelly, 64–65
rye pollen, 158

saffron, 83
sage, 158–59
sandalwood, 205–6
sarsaparilla, 159–161
sauerkraut, 83
saw palmetto, 161–63
schisandra, 163–4
selegiline, *see* deprenyl

self-esteem, 218–225
  and poor body image, 14–15
sensate focusing, 228–29
sepia, 185
serotonin, 9
sesame seeds, 84
sex drive
  men – boost your, 248–58
  women – boost your, 258–68
sexual
  abuse, 31
  memory, 10–11
shrimps, 84
Siberian ginseng, 164–67
sleep
  lack of, 16–17
smoking, 19
soy bean extracts, 67–68
St Johns Wort, *see* hypericum
staphysagria, 185
star anise, *see* aniseed
strawberries, 84
stress, 15–16
sulphur, 185–86
sunshine
  lack of, 31

testosterone, 7–9, 96–100
  from wild yam, 100
therapy
  transactional analysis, 238–39
  behaviour, 239